What They Don't Tell You About *Menopause*

A Gynecologist's Unofficial Guide to Premenopausal, Perimenopausal, and Postmenopausal Life

Dr. Heather L. Johnson

WHAT THEY DON'T TELL YOU ABOUT MENOPAUSE: A GYNECOLOGIST'S UNOFFICIAL GUIDE TO PREMENOPAUSAL, PERIMENOPAUSAL, AND POSTMENOPAUSAL LIFE

1405 SW 6th Avenue • Ocala, Florida 34471 • Phone 352-622-1825 • Fax 352-622-1875
Website: www.atlantic-pub.com • Email: sales@atlantic-pub.com
SAN Number: 268-1250

Library of Congress Control Number: 2020919132

Printed in the United States

PROJECT MANAGER: Crystal Edwards
INTERIOR LAYOUT AND JACKET DESIGN: Nicole Sturk

Dedication

This book is dedicated to Dr. Paula McKrisky a.k.a. the guru—one of the kindest, most knowledgeable and dedicated physicians and individuals I have ever had the pleasure to know, work with and learn from. Her retirement from the field of gynecology will be a tremendous loss to all, but her wisdom will live on. Thank you, Paula, for all you have done for so many.

Table of Contents

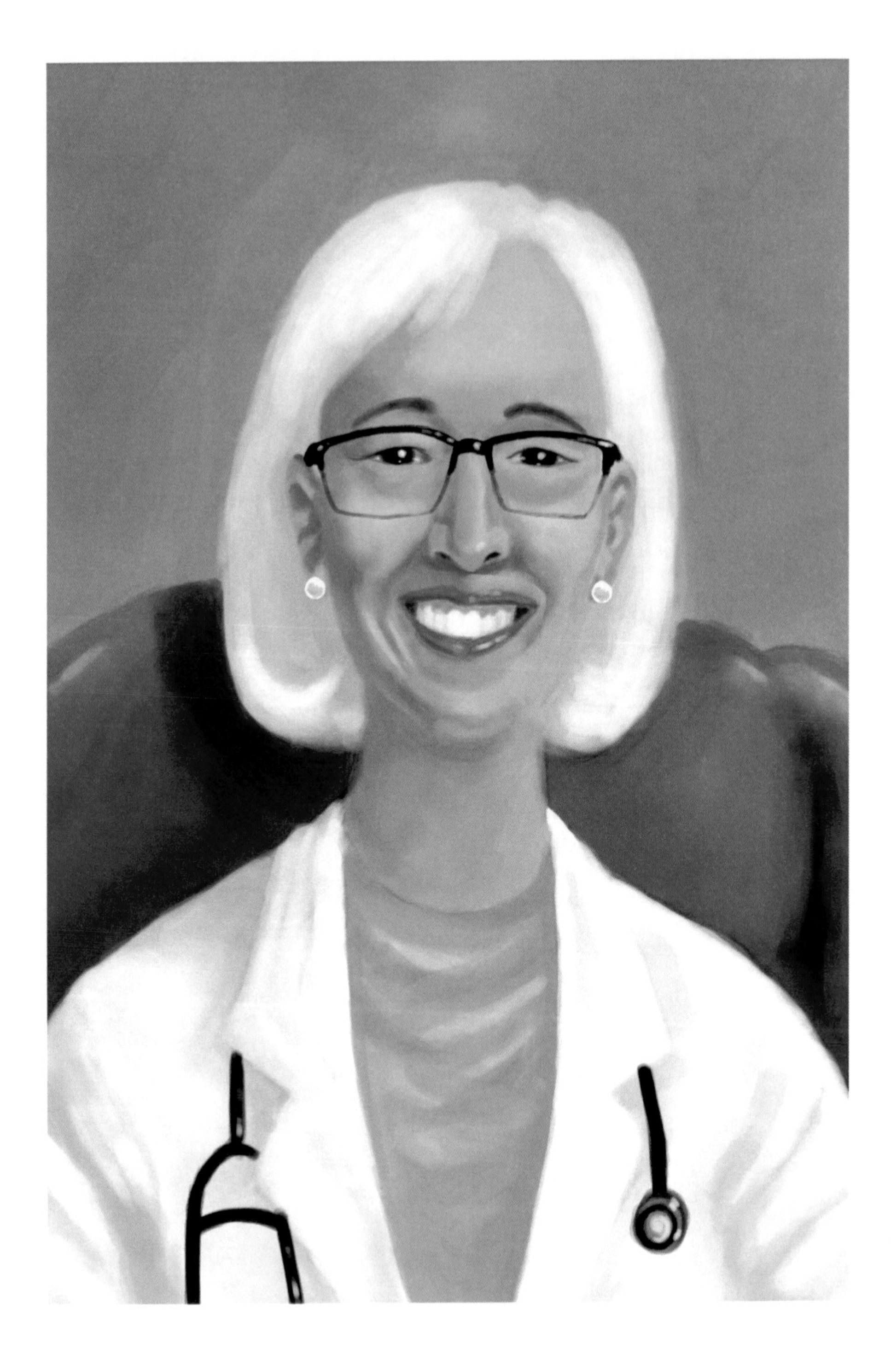

Introduction

Did you know that four species of whales—the orca, the beluga, the narwhal and the pilot—are the only mammals besides humans to go through menopause?[1] All other mammals reproduce until they die. Of course, this means they die in the prime of their lives, which is something most humans are not interested in doing. Did you know that the average caveman lived only 25 years? (It's true this number is skewed by the extremely high infant mortality rate, but still, not very long.) Did you know that in biblical times most did not live beyond their 30s, dying from childbirth, infectious diseases, malnutrition, etc.? It was not until the 1900s that a significant number of women began to live long enough to experience menopause. Now, most women live into their 70s and 80s, a mixed but welcome blessing.[2]

This relatively new phenomenon means that women are faced with a challenge that our ancestors did not experience: estrogen deficiency. This exposes us to increasing risks for osteoporosis, heart disease, elevated cholesterol, vaginal dryness with resulting pain related to intercourse, mood swings, hot flashes, and other debilitating conditions. Until the baby boomers came of age, many of these issues were rarely discussed amongst women, in medical journals, or on television. Even the word "menopause" was often uttered in hushed tones, as if it were something about which to

1. Quartz Daily, 2018
2. Wikipedia, 2020

be ashamed. I remember being chastised by a woman on the DC metro in the early 1990s for carrying a bag advertising the North American Menopause Society (NAMS). Fortunately, that has all changed. There is a wealth of information (and, sadly, misinformation) about this period of life, which is now accepted as a normal stage of life rather than a disorder. My hope is that this book will offer practical, fact-based, supportive information for women in their mid or late menstrual lives in order to assist them on their journey.

The average age of menopause in the United States is 51 with most women having their last menstrual period between 48–52. The age you enter menopause is determined by factors including family history and ethnicity. For instance, Japanese women generally enter menopause at a later age, while Hispanic women tend to enter at an earlier age. Smokers often experience menopause at an earlier age. Women who have had hysterectomies, even if their ovaries were preserved, and women with previous chemotherapy also tend to enter menopause earlier. How you experience menopause is also variable. Family history and race play roles, with African Americans experiencing more hot flashes and night sweats than others. Lifestyle factors such as diet, exercise, obesity, and smoking also weigh into the formula.[3]

In my late 30s and early 40s, I started giving presentations about menopause to women (and any men who were interested). While talking about the consequences, I was certain that the unfortunate changes associated with menopause would not happen to me. I was also certain before having a baby that I would not be THAT woman who had painful labors, excessive weight gain, mood swings, etc. Then I got pregnant and gained an unpublishable amount of weight, had previously unexperienced emotional highs and lows, and got stretch marks! I accepted an epidural early in labor and ended up needing a cesarean section for a baby weighing over nine pounds. I had postpartum depression and failed to lose weight in a timely fashion (but ultimately did). While I was humbled by my pregnancy

3. Practice Bulletin, 2014

experiences, I was absolutely thrilled (and still am) with the amazing individuals I brought into this world and into my life.

Unfortunately, my humbled self did not learn from these life experiences. As I approached menopause, I was absolutely certain I would not be THAT women who suffered the consequences of estrogen deficiency. I had a few "warm surges" early on and was certain that I was strong and special—and then reality hit. I experienced literally dozens of hot flashes. (And let me tell you, that is a misnomer. They are not just "flashes." They are intense and prolonged surges of overwhelming heat that can make an otherwise sane woman want to strip naked and stand in front of an open freezer, something most people do not want to see a 50 something year old woman do!) I would be literally drenched with sweat several times an hour. (My dry cleaner loved it.)

I distinctly remember having dinner one night with my husband and son, who was home on vacation from law school. During the course of the meal, I repeated the following refrains: Remove sweater. Put scrunchie on hair to make a ponytail. Turn on battery operated fan. Wipe sweat. Turn off fan. Put sweater back on. Remove scrunchie. Repeat. On the third iteration, I caught the look between my husband and my son. That look said, "If you say anything, you will surely die!" This eventually led to a family intervention of sorts. "You need to do something about this." I, of course, felt that I had everything under control.

A couple of weeks later, I was performing a scheduled cesarean section on the wife of one of my colleagues. The sweating started, per routine, after the uterine incision was closed. By the time I was closing the skin, I needed to ask the surgical assistant to wipe my brow because my sweat was about to drop into the incision. When I finished the procedure, my scrub suit was saturated. It looked as if I had gone for a swim. That was it — I had had enough of the "flashes!" The very next day, when I got to the office, I went to the sample cabinet and took out some estrogen replacement and started it. Within a few days, I was pretty much symptom free. Although I had an occasional hot flash, I was a happy camper for the next five years.

At that time, my daughter, an internal medicine physician, pleaded with me to stop taking hormone replacement therapy because my mother had breast cancer at the age of 69. (She went on to live into her late 80s cancer-free by the way.) She recommended what most internists recommend: an antidepressant. I advised her that would not be sufficient, but she persisted, so I tried it. True to form, the antidepressant provided what I will call a "20 percent discount." The flashes were either 20 percent less frequent or 20 percent less bothersome. Fortunately, at this point, my symptoms were less frequent and less severe, so I continued. To this day (after approximately 18 years of this flashing nonsense), I still get several dozen a week. Yes, they are more manageable, and yes, in general, they are less severe. But the bottom line is, they persist.

The good news is that most women do not suffer as long or as severely as I have or do. Most have 6–12 months of symptoms at worst, and some do not have any at all. I'm guessing the goddesses of menopause have been playing with me to better help me understand my patients, family, and friends. Hence this book, which is for all menopausal women. Those with hot flashes, vaginal dryness, pain with intercourse, bone loss, joint pain, heart disease, weight gain, (OK, so there aren't any of those!) increased abdominal girth, emotional symptoms, and/or fertility issues—and those without. In other words, this book is for all women in their 40s, 50s, and beyond along with those who may be experiencing symptoms in their 30s due to a hysterectomy or premature ovarian insufficiency, previously termed premature menopause.

As I shared with readers in my first book, *What They Don't Tell You About Having A Baby: An Obstetrician's Unofficial Guide to Preconception, Pregnancy, and Postpartum Life*, I have been truly blessed with my career choice and by my amazing patients who have taught me much more than I could ever have gleaned from books and journals. Their support and requests for a compilation of what I have learned about the journey to and through this phase of life have encouraged me to write this book. What follows should not be viewed so much as an official manual for menopause; there are plenty of books that cover this. Rather, it should be looked upon as a collection of the real conversations I have had with my patients, colleagues, and friends, and of the many experiences and lessons learned (including my own) along the way, as well as with some of my bite sized advice and information that I refer to as my "Dr. J's Pearls." The intent is to pass along my observations and medical insights in the hope they might be helpful to patients and providers.

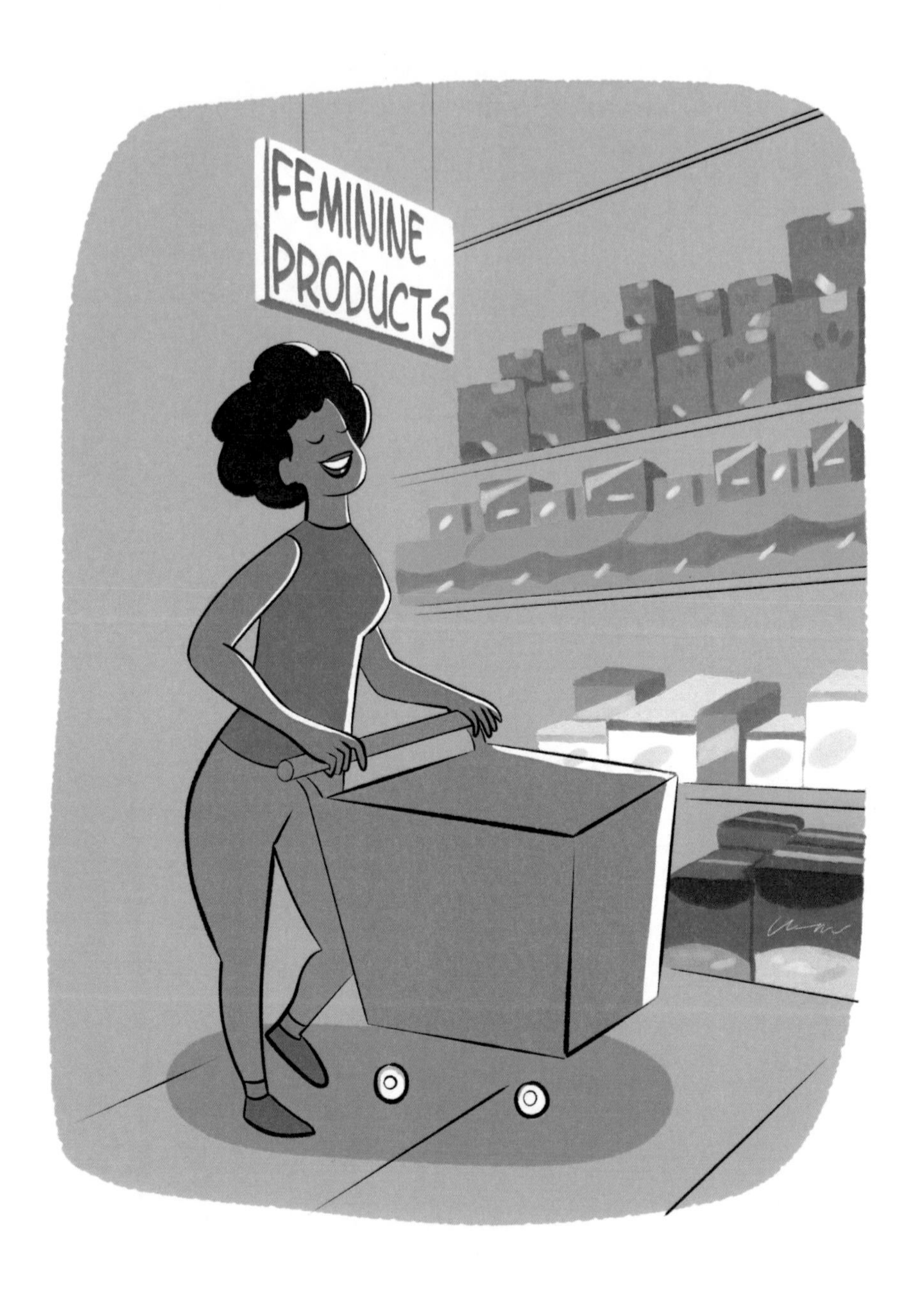
FEMININE
PRODUCTS

Part One

Premenopause

What exactly is premenopause? Technically speaking, a five-year-old, a teenager, and a 30-year-old are all PRE, or before, menopause, but that is not the true meaning of the word. Premenopause is used to describe women in their later reproductive years, or early to mid-40s, who are still having regular menstrual cycles. There are some subtle hormonal changes occurring, but they are not symptomatic. They do not have hot flashes. They are, with decreasing ability, capable of reproducing. They are not yet old, but definitely no longer young. They are full-on adult women in what many would consider the prime of their lives: vital and productive forces of nature, mothers, mentors, leaders, and builders with experience bordering on wisdom. (You have to be a bit older to claim that one fully!) This chapter will focus on some of the changes that can be expected during this amazing time of life.

Menstrual Cycles and Bleeding Issues

First, let's define normal. The typical woman who is not on hormonal birth control menstruates every 24–38 days with the average being 27–28 days. (There are women who swear that they bleed every 28 days exactly, but numerous studies of those who claim that regularity generally demonstrate an average of 25–29 days with the average being 28.) For most women, flow generally lasts 5–7 days. Average blood loss during a cycle is less than or equal to 80 ml[4] or 2.7 oz. (There are 8 ounces in a cup.) If you ask the average gynecologist what they mean by heavy bleeding, they will likely say soaking through a pad or a tampon an hour for more than a few hours, but the more official definition is bleeding in an amount or quantity that interferes with a woman's life. Mid-cycle spotting occurs in a minority of women at the time of ovulation. This may be due to the sudden estrogen/progesterone imbalance and is not considered pathological.

Normal premenstrual symptoms, known as molimina, include uterine cramping, tender breasts, fluid retention, mood swings, constipation, and increase in appetite. Most women experience some form of this if not on hormonal contraception. When these symptoms become more severe and interfere with everyday life, they are referred to as premenstrual syndrome (PMS). Extreme cases are classified as premenstrual dysphoric disorder (PMDD). Something that I have noticed in many patients in their 40s, especially those in their later 40s, is either the worsening of PMS symptoms or their appearance for the first time. Women complain they can see themselves becoming raging wild people over minor incidents. I can't tell you that I understand the physiology behind this, but it does occur frequently. Lifestyle changes can be helpful at this point. Birth control pills often work, especially if taken in a continuous manner to avoid cycles at all. For some women, increased aerobic activity or calcium intake prior to and during menses works to lessen the severity of their pain and discomfort. Certain antidepressants taken in continuous or cyclic fashion can be helpful as well. Everyone is different. Many times, the assurance that this often happens at their age is enough. Reassurance and tracking closely to be aware when they might be vulnerable and should avoid contact with humans, at least the ones they love or could fire them, is often enough.

Along with the decrease in quality and quantity of eggs as women age often comes a change in menstrual bleeding. While I've not seen this described in any medical journals, many of my patients have observed the following, which I have now come to define as "age appropriate." Their cycles used to be 28 days on average, lasting 5–7 days with moderate flow throughout.

4. UpToDate, 2019

Sometime in their early 40s, they begin to notice that their cycles start getting closer together, maybe averaging 25 days. The flow is often extremely heavy (described by some as a crime scene requiring wings, overnight pads, and embarrassing checks to the chair you just got up from at work) and/or that the blood has changed from a thinner to a thicker consistency, like giant clotty globs. That lasts for a day or two and then peters out to light or minimal staining for the remaining 3–4 days, just enough to require protection. After years of ordering various tests (e.g., blood counts, sonograms and uterine biopsies) for my patients in their 40s for what sounded to me to be abnormal menstrual cycles, I ultimately found that the majority were absolutely normal. They were not anemic because the heavy flow was for only a day or two followed by light bleeding, with the average loss likely to be the same as for those who bled consistently each day. Once reassured by the normalcy and predictability of their situation, most opted to do nothing further than closely monitor their cycles. Others selected options like intrauterine devices (IUDs) or birth control pills, a topic I discuss later in this section.

Absent this exception, any irregular bleeding after the age of 40 needs to be evaluated, because women over 40 are at increased risk for developing uterine cancer or atypical endometrial (cells lining the uterine cavity) hyperplasia, it's precursor. Both often present with irregular bleeding. If you find that your cycles are suddenly becoming heavier or longer or if you have unpredictable bleeding in between your periods, talk with your provider. In many cases, a benign cause such as a polyp or fibroid or no structural abnormality at all will be found and options of observation, change in birth control, or outpatient surgical procedures will be discussed to control the symptoms. The workup to exclude abnormal cells can include a sonogram to evaluate the endometrial stripe, or thickness of the lining of the uterus. A uterine lining that is too thick can suggest buildup of abnormal cells. Another option would be to have an office procedure called an endometrial biopsy (EMB) to obtain cells from the uterine cavity for pathologic evaluation. The procedure can be uncomfortable, especially if you haven't had a baby or are postmenopausal, but it is tolerable. For most women, it's less uncomfortable than having an IUD inserted.

There are many other causes for abnormal uterine bleeding. For the purposes of this book, I will concentrate on those that tend to present themselves in mid-life.

Uterine Fibroids or Leiomyomas

Uterine fibroids or leiomyomas are benign tumors comprised of muscle cells and fibrous connective tissue. They are common, affecting about a quarter of reproductive-aged women, and occur with increasing frequency as women age. Uterine fibroids or leiomyomas are prevalent in the African American population, almost the rule rather than the exception, and you are more likely to develop them if your mother had them. The good news is because they are estrogen dependent, they stop growing after menopause. In fact, any increase in fibroid size after menopause is cause for investigation.

For most women, fibroids are not a problem and are generally found incidentally during a pelvic exam or sonogram. However, for some the fibroids grow large enough to cause a noticeable bulge in their abdomen that resembles anywhere between a 10–20-week pregnancy. Small fibroids on the anterior surface of the uterus can keep the bladder from filling normally, resulting in a frequent need to urinate. Larger and posterior ones can impede the flow of urine from the kidney to the bladder. The most common effect of fibroids and the one likely to lead to medical or surgical intervention is the development of heavy and/or prolonged menstrual bleeding that can result in anemia, because the body cannot keep up with the loss of blood through diet or supplemental iron. Options for treatment include hormonal birth control like oral contraceptives (OCs), Depo-Provera, and progesterone containing IUDs along with myomectomy, or removal of the fibroids leaving the uterus intact, uterine artery embolization (UAE), and hysterectomy. Please check with your provider for more detailed discussion of the best options for you.

Uterine Polyps

Uterine polyps, or endometrial polyps, are made from the tissue lining the uterine cavity, or endometrium, and are generally benign soft tissue growths that become more prevalent with age. They typically present with bleeding in between menstrual cycles and/or with heavier menstrual bleeding. If symptomatic, these polyps can be removed in a procedure called a polypectomy that is performed through the vagina. Some anesthesia is needed, so the surgery is often performed in an operating room or outpatient surgical center. The only down time is the day of surgery—you can go back to life the next day.

Adenomyosis

Adenomyosis is a condition where the endometrial glands, which normally line the uterine cavity, grow into the surrounding muscular tissue of the uterus and cause swelling of the surrounding tissue, resulting in an enlarged, boggy uterus. This condition is more common in women who have had babies and can result in periods that are heavier, longer, and more painful than normal. The diagnosis is generally suspected on ultrasound. Treatment options are similar to those for fibroids except that adenomyosis cannot be removed in bulk because of its diffuse involvement in the uterine wall.

Fertility Issues

The ovaries develop in a female fetus by the end of the first trimester. By 20 weeks (five months), they contain 6–7 million immature eggs. This is the most a female will ever have—no more new eggs form after this. From this point on, there is a steady decrease in the number of eggs as some mature to a point and then degenerate in a process called atresia. By the time a female is born, she has only one million of the original 6–7 million eggs left. This process continues in childhood so that only 300,000 remain by puberty. During reproductive years, under the influence of various hormones, some of the eggs will finish their maturational process and be released mid-cycle. If fertilized, pregnancy ensues. The average female will only actually release 300–400 mature eggs in her lifetime. So yes, we are all very special and unique—1 in 6–7 million![5]

5. Rogel Cancer Center, 2020

As women age, the number of remaining eggs decreases. At age 37, a woman has approximately 25,000 eggs left. At 51, that number is about 1,000, and more of the remaining eggs become abnormal, thus decreasing the chance for pregnancy and increasing the chance for chromosomal abnormalities such as Down syndrome.[6] As you can see from the chart, the risk for Down syndrome from ages 20–24 is 1/1400. By age 40, that risk is 1/100 with the risk for all chromosomal abnormalities reaching 1/63. Many, if not most, of these types of pregnancies result in a spontaneous miscarriage.

Along with declining egg number and quality, the risks of primary gynecologic disorders such as fibroids (benign, muscular tumors of the uterus), uterine polyps (benign fleshy growths in the uterine cavity), endometriosis (growth of uterine lining cells outside of the uterine cavity onto other pelvic organs), and pelvic infection increase with time, confounding the already decreasing fertility rate.

I have been known to say that teenagers can stand downwind of sperm and get pregnant, 40-year-olds, not so much. As discussed in the Introduction of this book, nature did not plan for humans to live as long as we now do. Thus, it made sense for women to stop reproducing long enough before their death that they could raise their children. Fertility is greatest in the late teens and early twenties. With increasing nutrition, adolescence and menarche (the age at which females start to menstruate) has occurred at younger ages with the first period occurring between the ages of 10–16 in most developed nations—a mixed blessing since adolescent pregnancies are fraught with more complications. The fertility rate begins to drop gradually by about age 32. After 35, that drop becomes steeper, although most women can still conceive on their own until about 37 or 38. After that, the chances of needing assisted reproductive technology increases. Fertility rates decrease dramatically after 40, with each 6–12-month period associated with less likelihood of spontaneous pregnancy. A woman's chances of conceiving after trying for 3 months at age 25 are 18 percent; at age 30 are 16 percent; at age 35 are 12 percent; and at age 40 are 7 percent. Prior to 35, women are encouraged to try for pregnancy for a year before seeking

6. Healthline Parenthood, 2020

assistance. At 35, they are encouraged to do so after six months or sooner if they have been timing their ovulations. Women 40 and over are encouraged to seek help at the outset. [7]

Frequency of Down Syndrome Per Maternal Age

Age (years)	Frequency of Fetuses with Down Syndrome to Normal Fetuses at 16 weeks of pregnancy	Frequency of Live Births of Babies with Down Syndrome to Normal Births
15-19	----	1/1250
20-24	----	1/1400
25-29	----	1/1100
30-31	----	1/900
32	----	1/750
33	1/420	1/625
34	1/325	1/500
35	1/250	1/350
36	1/200	1/275
37	1/150	1/225
38	1/120	1/175
39	1/100	1/140
40	1/75	1/100
41	1/60	1/85
42	1/45	1/65
43	1/35	1/50
44	1/30	1/40
45 and older	1/20	1/25

The numbers are approximated and rounded. Using this data, geneticists have set the number separating low-risk from high-risk at 1/250.

There is a difference in frequencies between 16 weeks and time of birth due to spontaneous miscarriages of pregnancies with Down syndrome between these times.

For information on risks of more detailed situations (such as translocation or mothers who have had previous babies with Down syndrome, see Dr. Paul Benke's essay on Risk and Recurrence of Down syndrome.

Reference for the above table: Hook EB. JAMA 249:2034-2038, 1983. [8]

7. Healthline Parenthood, 2020
8. Hook, E. 1983

While unassisted pregnancy beyond 45 is possible, it occurs in less than 5 percent of women with a high miscarriage rate. There are many reports about women in their 50s having babies—some substantiated, others not. The vast majority of women in their 50s and beyond having babies today do so with donor eggs from younger women, even if they don't tell you that is the case. The oldest woman I ever delivered was 56 (with a donor egg, of course). She and her baby did quite well. I haven't seen her postpartum so I have no idea how she is handling motherhood in her 50s and 60s. That's a whole other story! Suffice it to say, fertility decreases as women age and decreases dramatically from the mid-30s on. Just because you are having regular periods does not mean that you are fertile. Options such as egg freezing, or fertility preservation, donor egg, and in vitro fertilization (IVF) exist and can result in a healthy baby and a healthy mom.

Many of my patients who are considering the timing of their pregnancy (e.g., they want to wait until after their wedding in a year; they want to finish their PhD thesis; they or their partner is in graduate school; they just bought a house; they just aren't ready) request that I order blood work to "check my fertility." These tests, Anti-Müllerian hormone (AMH), and the levels of follicle stimulating hormone (FSH) and estradiol on day three of their menstrual cycle are, in some ways, an indirect measure of your ovarian reserve. Levels in the normal range suggest that you have sufficient reserve and are, therefore, potentially fertile. Note that a normal value does not guarantee that you can get pregnant, just that your levels are in the normal range for people who can conceive. It is also only a snapshot in time. If it is normal this year, it may not be normal in another year. If it is abnormal, you might have to reconsider your timing or speak with a specialist about potentially freezing your eggs, otherwise known as fertility preservation, or using donor eggs. Note that day three FSH and estradiol can only be drawn if you are ovulating, which means they cannot be drawn while taking any form of hormonal birth control that suppresses ovulation such as the pill, the patch, the vaginal ring, or Depo-Provera. AMH can be drawn while taking these medications, but results are considered by some to be more reliable if you are off the pill for at least one cycle.

Less than 1 percent of women develop premature ovarian insufficiency (POI), which is basically early menopause. There are various reasons for this including family history, chromosomal abnormality, autoimmune disorders, or previous chemotherapy, but many of these situations are simply spontaneous. If you are concerned about this, please seek medical advice as early as possible.

Birth Control

While pregnancy becomes less likely as women grow older, age 40 is not the time to stop using birth control unless a pregnancy would be welcome. I have delivered far too many babies to women who thought they were too old to conceive because they were 40 or over.

The good news is that most birth control options available to younger women are also appropriate for women 40 and beyond. The exception is the birth control pill, which has been proven safe to use up to the age of 50 but should not be used in smokers over 35 or those with uncontrolled blood pressure due to the increased risk for cardiovascular disease. Another potential exclusion for older women is natural family planning, since cycles become less predictable as one approaches menopause making this option less reliable.

Barrier Methods

Barrier methods of any kind are appropriate during the last decade of reproductive life. Along with decreasing libido and/or frequency of intercourse, which I will talk about later, this often turns out to be a good solution. Options include condoms with or without spermicides, diaphragms (an oldie but goodie), and the contraceptive sponge, if you can find it. Downsides to the use of these options include potential allergic reactions to ingredients or materials and possible increase in the occurrence of yeast infections and/or urinary tract infections. The sponge and diaphragm can be inserted in advance and thus are less likely to interfere with spontaneity. Condoms must be placed when the penis is erect, something that can be a bit disruptive.

Hormonal Birth Control

Depo-Provera, a highly effective form of birth control, is still offered but not very popular these days given the other available options. It is a shot that has to be given every three months, which many may find inconvenient, but tends to take your periods away, which most find a pleasant side effect. The biggest drawback for most women is that the shots often lead to significant weight gain. Skinny teenagers can take the shots with no repercussions, but overweight, especially older overweight women, frequently find they put on a distressing amount of weight, often to the tune of 10-15 pounds.

Nexplanon is a progesterone implant placed in the arm. It offers excellent protection for three years and does not contain estrogen. However, bleeding patterns are not very predictable. Some women have no bleeding the entire three years, some have regular but lighter cycles, and some have unpredictable bleeding either with infrequent cycles or unpredictable spotting.

Birth control pills, also known as oral contraceptive pills (OCs or OCPs), as well as the vaginal ring and the birth control patch are excellent options for those who don't smoke or have significant medical problems that put them at increased risk for cardiovascular disease. The pill tends to make your periods lighter or even absent. Cramps generally improve or disappear altogether. The best benefit is that, as you get closer to menopause, you will likely not experience the hot flashes and night sweats your friends are experiencing, because the estrogen levels from the pill are high enough to overcome that. In most cases, you can safely take the pill to age 50. Hopefully, when you stop taking it, you will be on the other side of menopause and have escaped those often-distressing symptoms.

Intrauterine devices (IUDs) are another effective form of birth control. There are two types of IUDs available – hormonal, which contain progesterone, and non-hormonal, which contain copper. The copper IUD (e.g., Paragard) is good for 10 years but tends to make your periods heavier with more cramping, an unwelcome side effect for many women. IUDs with progesterone (i.e., Mirena and Kyleena) last for five years or more, and the amount of progesterone released is significantly less than with birth control pills or Nexplanon. Most of the work is done in the uterine cavity, not in your bloodstream. They do not contain estrogen. The side effect is that many women, especially those who use Mirena or its generic equivalent, end up having no periods at all after a few months. While disturbing to some, it is a welcome relief to many women.

Medical Procedures

Permanent Sterilization

For women, having her partner get a vasectomy can be the easiest, most painless option—and a logical one for those who have had their uterus ripped asunder by a baby or two or three. It is effective as well with a failure rate of less than 1 percent. If you can work this out with your partner, good for you. However, in the years I have practiced, I have come to realize that there are really only two kinds of men—those who CAN have a vasectomy and those who CAN'T. It's really not a WILL or WON'T thing. It's connected somewhere in their male brains with that pesky Y chromosome. This is the one thing I've learned to let husbands/partners get away with in my years of practice. It is not rational. It does not depend on their education. It has nothing to do with whether they love you or not. Some men simply CAN'T. If you find that your husband/partner has been promising to see the urologist but has not ever actually done so, and two to three or more years have passed, let me tell you it's not going to happen. They will use condoms or go without sex before they will undergo the procedure.

Female sterilization is, of course, also an option. The upside is that it requires one procedure. Yes, there is a recovery time that may require up to a week off of work and perhaps two weeks without vigorous exercise. As with all medical procedures, there is the possibility of unexpected complications. However, nothing else has to be done after that. Though effective, there is a chance of ectopic pregnancy, which is when a pregnancy develops in the fallopian tube and could threaten your life. (The same is true for IUDs, by the way, which are as effective as permanent sterilization.) A difference today is that the recommended form of female sterilization is removal of the entire tube rather than just severing or "tying" it. This is because data shows that a good number of ovarian cancers actually start in the fimbriated terminal ends of the fallopian tube and spread to the ovary. Removing the tube removes that risk. Those with a family history of ovarian cancer may want to consider this option if they are not ready to have their ovaries removed. The pill, by the way, also decreases the risk for ovarian cancer. The longer you take it, the lower your risk.

Endometrial Ablation

Endometrial ablation is a procedure performed on some women for heavy bleeding. The lining of the uterine cavity (endometrium) is thinned considerably after ablation, making pregnancy difficult to attain. However, it should not be considered a form of birth control.

Hysterectomy

Without a uterus, pregnancy is not possible. However, if you retain your ovaries, your eggs can be used along with your partner's sperm in a gestational carrier. The baby will be genetically yours.

Sexually Transmitted Illnesses (STIs)

Many women assume, rightfully or not, that they cannot get pregnant after 40 and stop using condoms. If you are in a committed and mutually monogamous relationship, the decision should be based on your age, what else you may be doing for birth control, and/or whether or not an unplanned pregnancy would be a welcome surprise. Gone are the days, if they ever really existed, that most women could expect to have one sexual partner from marriage on through the rest of their lives. People get divorced. Spouses die. Spouses and partners can be unfaithful. While one of the most dreaded complications of a sexually transmitted illness (STI) is infertility as a result of gonorrhea or chlamydia infections and the development of pelvic inflammatory disease (PID), this is generally not a concern for women in their 40s and beyond. However, everyone wants to avoid the contraction of herpes, syphilis, hepatitis, and HIV/AIDs. I have seen far too many women in their 50s and 60s with these unexpected "gifts" from their partners, so please, have the talk. Do the testing. Use protection as indicated.

Human papilloma virus (HPV) is a sexually transmitted virus that causes cervical cancer. There are many strains of HPV, and most are considered low risk for leading to the development of abnormal cells, precancers, and cancers of the cervix. In addition to having a Pap test at your yearly check-up, your gynecologist may also offer testing for what are known as the high-risk HPV strains, or the ones more likely to lead to cervical cancer. Three strains—16, 18 and 45—are responsible for the majority of cervical cancers and precancers. If you test positive for these strains, you will be offered a procedure called a colposcopy where the cervix is evaluated using a microscope and samples of tissue are taken for laboratory evaluation. Follow-up or treatment will depend upon the extent of involvement. You should know that the current recommendations by the American College of Obstetricians and Gynecologists (ACOG) for the frequency of Pap smear testing are based on the assumption that exposure is far less in older women which, in most cases, is a reasonable one. While not a current recommendation, you might consider testing if you have recently become active again with a new partner, especially since older women tend to have more trouble eradicating the virus from their system than teenagers and those in their twenties, who generally clear it within six months to a year or two.

Gardasil 9 is a vaccine for HPV given to adolescent boys and girls to decrease their risk of getting HPV and, thus, their risk for getting cervical cancer. The HPV vaccine series comprises three shots for those over 15 (but only two shots for those aged 9 – 14): an initial one, a second shot two months later, and a third shot administered six months after the first one. Boys are treated because they are the vectors that transfer the virus to their partners. When initially introduced, the recommendation was that the vaccine be offered to people from age 13–26. That's because the initial testing was done on this age group, and the FDA would only approve its use in the population studied. That being said, I've never met a virus that carded an individual before entry. It can infect you whatever age you are. If you're eligible, not allergic to any of the ingredients, and have the means to do so, I would suggest you consider getting this vaccine. Fortunately, follow-up has now been long enough that FDA approval has been given for use in adults up to the age of 45. Unfortunately, as of this writing, many insurance companies have chosen not to cover the vaccine for women over

26, although some have shown responsibility and are choosing to extend coverage. Hopefully others will soon follow suit.

Please check with your insurance company before getting vaccinated so you are not caught by surprise bills afterward. The vaccine series is expensive, generally around $300 US each not including injection fees. Make a stink about it with your insurance if you need to. After all, it is approved by the FDA and should be covered even if it is not yet "usual and customary." If you are over 45, sadly, you are on your own now. You can get the shots but will likely have to pay for them out-of-pocket if you are becoming sexually active again and want protection.

Pelvic Relaxation and Pelvic Floor Strengthening

I am including this section in the premenopausal portion of the book not because it is that common in this age group but because it is the time that you can use your youthful muscles and abundant estrogen (except of course, while you are nursing) to strengthen the area and forestall major problems later in life. Any woman who has the "pleasure" of having a baby traverse her vaginal canal knows that her vagina is never the same after that. I once heard a male colleague say, "It's like putting a piece of chewed up gum back in the wrapper. It will fit, but it will never fit the same." I was outraged when I heard him say that but thought later about the analogy and came to the conclusion that it was a correct one. The ability of the vagina to contract down to its former size, shape, and strength is lost forever after the first baby. If you have had a vaginal delivery, especially one of a larger-than-average baby (greater than 7–8 pounds), you might notice the fit with intercourse, while still pleasurable, is not the same. Also, immediately postpartum when your estrogen levels are low from breastfeeding, you may well lose a little urine when you cough, sneeze, laugh, or run. Fortunately for most, this resolves within a few weeks or months. However, as you get closer to menopause, this problem may recur with increasing frequency and severity.

The most bothersome part of this relaxation is what is known as stress urinary incontinence (SUI). This occurs with increased abdominal pressure from things such as high-impact aerobic activity, laughing, sneezing, or coughing and results in the involuntary loss of urine. The tendency for this to occur is worsened by obesity, the number of babies you have, family history, smoking, and ethnicity, with non-Hispanic white women faring the worst. Aging, with its associated loss in muscle throughout the body and decreasing estrogen levels, makes the problem more common as you approach menopause and significantly worse afterwards.

Fortunately, there is something you can do about it. That is the performance of Kegel exercises, which means exercising the pelvic, or Kegel, muscles on a regular basis. This strengthens the pelvic floor and decreases the symptoms. The exercise is performed by tightening the muscles of the vagina and rectum for about 10 seconds and repeating about 10 times. The official recommendation is to do these three times a day. I have found that 10 times a day is more effective. Make a game of it. Every time your baby cries, do 10. Every time the phone rings, do 10. Every time your child yells "mommy," do 10. Every time you stop at a traffic light, do 10. Like any exercise, regularity and consistency provide better results. Just like an occasional sit up or abdominal crunch will not result in a tightened core, occasion Kegels will not prevent or forestall future symptoms.

If you are not certain how to do the exercise, try stopping your urine flow midstream in the way you would if the house suddenly caught on fire. Please though, do not do this on a regular basis because there is some thought this could lead to an increase in urinary tract infections. If you are doing it correctly, the only muscles you should be using are your vaginal and rectal ones. You should not notice any contractions in your abdomen, buttocks or thighs. One physical therapist described it as pretending you are holding in a soaking wet tampon and trying to keep from passing gas at the same time.

If you cannot accomplish this on your own, there are weighted vaginal cones that you can order online. Start with the lowest weight and try to keep it in your vagina for a certain period of time before moving up in weight and size. You can do this on your own or with a pelvic floor physical therapist who also has other tricks up her sleeve, such as biofeedback. After menopause, you may need to add vaginal estrogen to your regimen to help maintain muscle strength in this area.

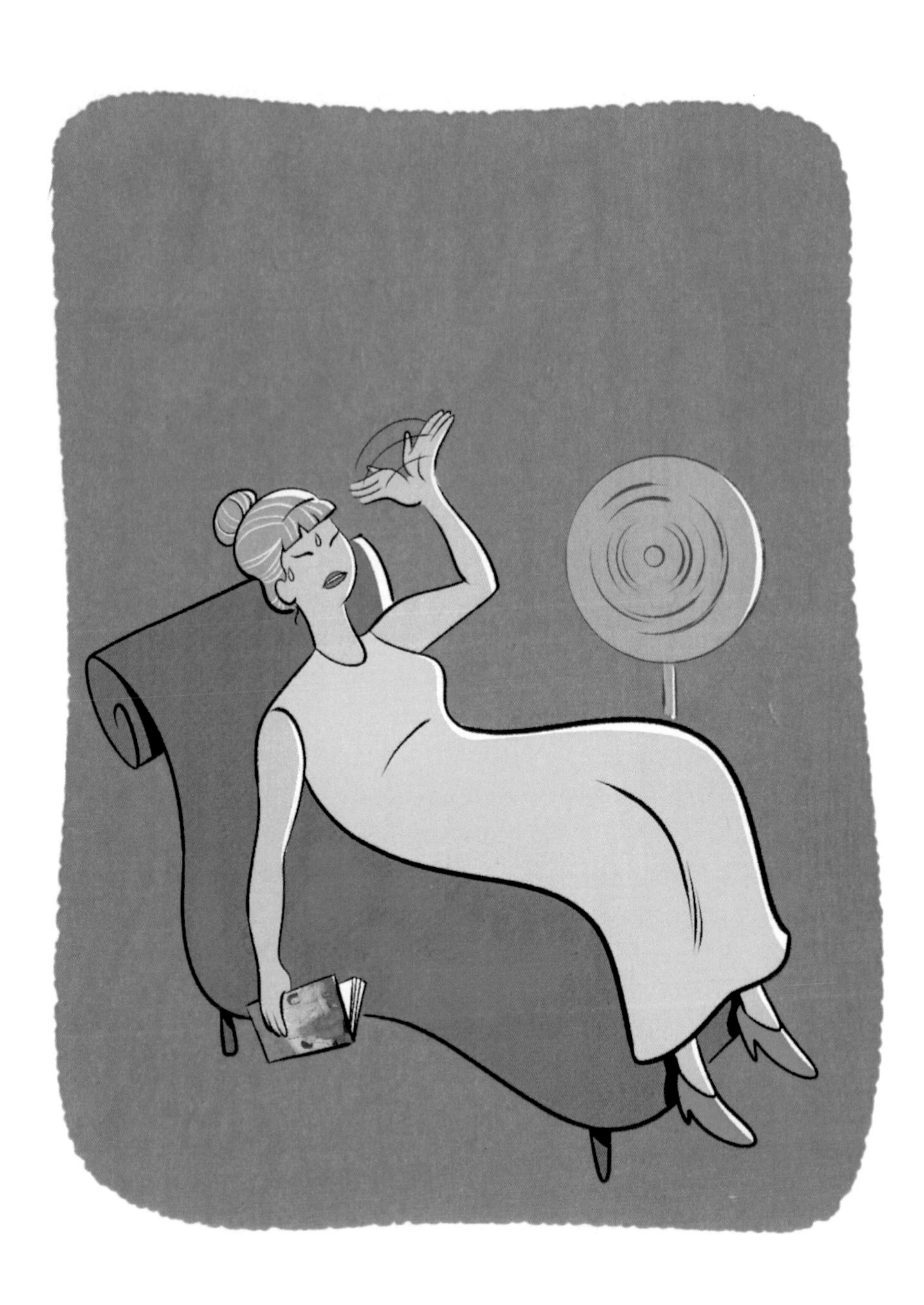

Part Two

Perimenopause or Climacteric

Perimenopause, also known as the climacteric, is literally the time around menopause that marks the end of the reproductive phase of life. It typically begins in the mid to late 40s and can precede the last menstrual period by a few months to a couple of years. The average age in the US for the last menstrual period is 51, but the range can be from 48–52.

This is where things start to get real for women, their partners, their families, and their coworkers as changes begin to occur, including menstrual cycle irregularities, hot flashes, sleep disturbances, muscular/joint aches and pain, and mood swings.

During this time, few eggs remain, and many of them are abnormal. Therefore, successful ovulations are less frequent and result in less predictability in your cycle. Your period may be a few weeks late followed by another period a couple of weeks later. The blood flow becomes less consistent and less predictable. You may start to have night sweats, hot flashes, insomnia, and mood swings for a few days or weeks and then feel fine. A week or two later, you get a period.

Average estrogen levels are lower during this time frame. As a result, your body produces a hormone called FSH, or follicle stimulating hormone, to stimulate the release of an egg. The closer you get to menopause, the lower your overall estrogen levels are and the higher your FSH needs to be to induce an ovulation. Once an egg is released and the estrogen levels rise, the FSH returns to normal. This is why testing for FSH in the perimenopausal period is not always helpful, since it depends upon where you are in your cycle. After menopause, the level is continuously elevated over the premenopausal levels. How long a woman remains perimenopausal varies considerably, ranging from a few months to a few years.

Bleeding Irregularities

An extremely small percentage of blessed women recall that they had normal cycles until they had no cycles at all. A larger number experience a few months of missed cycles followed by one long and murderous episode of bleeding before they cease having periods. The rest will experience changes in their cycles for anywhere for six months to a few years prior to the final cessation of menses. They may have anywhere from a handful to more than monthly cycles with less and less predictability in terms of flow, duration, and severity of symptoms such as fluid retention, constipation, breast tenderness, and mood swings. It is important at this time to keep track of your bleeding; while the likely cause is hormonal imbalance with less frequent or proper ovulations from older eggs, there are a number of other causes for irregular bleeding. Fortunately, most of these are benign but could result in the need for treatment. (For more detailed information, please see the section on Bleeding Irregularities in Part Two of this book.) The occurrence of uterine cancer increases with age and is a concern whenever there is unpredictable bleeding; this must be ruled out, because early treatment often results in a complete cure.

Vasomotor Symptoms a.k.a. Hot Flashes and Night Sweats

At least 80 percent of all women report some degree of vasomotor symptoms in the years preceding and following their last menstrual period. The mean duration of moderate to severe symptoms has been reported in some studies to be up to 4.9 years. Nine percent of women report symptoms up to the age of 72.[9] A biologist patient of mine once asked me what the evolutionary advantage of hot flashes was. I had no answer other than, perhaps, the capricious and whimsical will of the goddesses of chaos and disorder? While changing hormone levels clearly have something to do with it, their exact role is still not completely understood. Clearly, it is not the total lack of estrogen, otherwise five-year-old girls and 90-year-old women and all men would have them. (Imagine how challenging it would be to live in a household if everyone, regardless of their age or gender, were having hot flashes!) Studies discuss a potential resetting of the thermoregulatory zone and/or other complicated central physiologic mechanisms, which are way beyond the scope of this book. Suffice it to say that they exist.

There do appear to be racial and ethnic differences, with Asian women experiencing less and African American women more. It is not certain whether this is related to lifestyle issues such as diet and weight, genetic components, or both or none. Family history plays a role as well.[10] However, my mother was either an amazing actress or my two sisters and I are spontaneous mutants, since we've all had (and still have) our share of unwanted symptoms but we don't remember seeing our mother ever have a hot flash. In fact, my older sister started having sweats in her early 40s, long before any irregularities in her cycles. At the time, she had just started working as a school nurse in a high school that had a higher-than-average rate of students with tuberculosis (TB). She had such powerful symptoms that she got herself tested for TB before she finally realized that the "attacks" were related to menopause. I can identify with that, because the first time I had a serious night sweat, I dreamt that I had malaria. When I woke to wet sheets and pajamas, I knew it was a night sweat—and I was only 46 years old. Other factors such as obesity, smoking, and reduced physical activity can also affect the frequency and severity of hot flashes.[11]

Vasomotor symptoms can affect sleep and/or sleep quality. Those who are awakened by sweats several times a night fully understand why they are

9. UpToDate, 2020
10. UpToDate, 2020
11. UpToDate, 2020

fatigued the next day, but some do not experience symptoms severe enough to wake in a sweat. They may simply find themselves awakening many times at night for no apparent reason, at times with their heart beating faster than normal. This is because the sweat was not enough to register as one. They may also sleep through the night but toss and turn due to what I call "subliminal sweats." Many menopausal women complain of waking at 3 or 4 o'clock in the morning for no obvious reason. Be assured that millions of other women are awake at the same time wondering why. All of these changes can lead to or aggravate preexisting mood swings, anxiety, or depression.

Fortunately for most women, these symptoms are either short lived and/or mild. However, a significant minority have symptoms severe enough to seek treatment. When they occur with enough frequency and severity, they can lead to bothersome sleep disturbances which can result in fatigue, lethargy and mood swings—sort of like having a nursing infant that keeps you up all night. These disruptive symptoms can also interfere with everyday functions. It's difficult to keep a poker face at an office meeting if beads of sweat are rolling down your face and your blouse is drenched with sweat. I distinctly remember seeing one of my favorite reporters on the morning news break into a sweat with the cameras aimed directly at her face. Believe me, knowing that is happening only leads to more sweating. I felt for her and will love her to this day for the way she handled it, although I am certain she was mortified. So, what to do?

Most women can predict the onset of some of their symptoms. They may note that red wine or spicy foods can induce them. Stress or rushing can certainly do that for many. Sometimes they come at predictable times, such as after your morning shower, when you get into the car to go to work, or just before bed. Often doing things like sipping cold water, slowing down, or wearing layered clothing that can be removed easily helps. Turtlenecks are a no-no at this time—you may think they'll help hide the sweat running down your neck, but trust me, you'll regret having any extra fabric touching parts of your skin when a flash happens! Sleeping with one foot out of the covers helps a lot of women. Ceiling fans can become your next BFF. Sleeping naked on a beach towel also keeps you from the chills that arise after you soak your pajamas and sheets with sweat. Partners, you are going to need to step up now because your wife or partner is truly suffering. Complaining that you are cold when she sets the air conditioner at 60 degrees does nothing to alleviate her symptoms. Put on an extra blanket and be glad it's not you having those "attacks."

Regular exercise is touted to help, although I distinctly remember getting hot flashes in the middle of Bikram yoga classes, which are done in a room with a temperature of 105 degrees Fahrenheit. So much for that idea! As usual, gynecologists advise that women eat right, exercise regularly, avoid stress, and lose weight. All of these things are great in general; like chicken soup, it couldn't hurt. But I must say, for most it's like the Wizard of Oz telling Dorothy to get the Wicked Witch of the West's broomstick. No way was she going to do that, but she couldn't go home until she did.

OK, so we can agree that everyone should lead a healthy lifestyle, but what if that doesn't work, work enough, or simply doesn't happen? There are a number of over-the-counter treatments and alternative medical options that have been touted. Most have mixed reviews at best, are based on small studies with less than rigorous scientific standards and are generally not officially recommended by medical experts based on the evidence or lack thereof. However, these treatments and alternative options are not likely to be harmful if taken in appropriate amounts and, at worst, could have a beneficial placebo effect.

Chronic Pain: Muscular/Joint Aches and Pains and Migraine Headaches

A significant portion of my patients complains of either an increase or decrease in chronic pain at or around menopause. Most of my patients observe a significant reduction in the frequency and severity of migraines at this time. Many with chronic pain and/or joint or muscular aches and pains—whether or not they are related to conditions such as chronic fatigue syndrome, rheumatoid arthritis, or connective tissue diseases—notice an increase in their symptoms at and around menopause. While it is difficult to determine which of their symptoms are due to menopause or simply aging, a trial of hormone replacement therapy (HRT) may be useful at this time to determine if you are one of those lucky few who experience relief by this addition to your regimen.

Treatment Options

Botanical Plant-Based a.k.a. Natural Supplements

Health food stores, supermarkets, and online options for treating menopausal symptoms are numerous. Most are based on naturally occurring substances with the touted ability to limit or eliminate symptoms related to menopause. Unfortunately, while popular, many of these substances have not been well studied, and claims for success are often based on small sample sizes and anecdotal data.

Isoflavones and phytoestrogens are plant-based pseudo estrogens, meaning their structure is similar to estrogen, and they act in some ways like estrogen in the body. They can be found in things like soy, red clover, linseed, sesame seeds, fava beans, chickpeas, oats, and barley. There are a few studies that demonstrate effectiveness in reducing the number or severity of hot flashes but not night sweats. Most large studies, however, fail to demonstrate a statistically significant impact. St. John's wort, gingko biloba, evening primrose oil, vitamin E, ginseng, and DHEA have similar claims and limitations. For most of the above, taking them is not likely to result in harm other than to your wallet. These pseudo estrogens do all have a large placebo effect—upwards of 50 percent—but if they can get you through the night, they may be worth considering.

Please note that black cohosh taken in large amounts can cause liver toxicity. Dong quai in large amounts can increase the risk of bleeding when paired with Coumadin (Warfarin), an anticoagulant (blood thinner) medication taken by many people who are at an increased risk for blood clot formation.[12] Please be sure to talk to your doctor or pharmacist before introducing any new supplements or medication, as they all have potential

12. UpToDate, 2020

side effects, can cause allergic reactions and, as noted above, may interact positively or negatively with your other medications.

If you are going to try any of these options, I would suggest that you experiment with one at a time and give it a couple of months. If you take more than one at a time and have either improvement or side effects, you won't know which supplement/medication is responsible. Also, because symptoms can wax and wane during perimenopause, it's best you take it through what would have been a couple of cycles to see if it is just coincidence that you started to feel better after taking it.

Complementary and Alternative Medicine (CAM)

CAM health care approaches are not typically part of conventional/traditional Western medical care. Some examples include acupuncture, reflexology, cognitive behavioral therapy, hypnosis, and mindfulness training. These options oftentimes lack supportive, rigorous scientific evidence of their efficacy. However, women who are especially sensitive and/or allergic to medications and hormones can sometimes benefit from these modalities. If you choose any of these methods, please be sure to let your medical provider know so he or she can place it in your medical record.

Prescription Medicines: Clonidine and Gabapentin

At this point, I would like to mention two medications that come up whenever alternatives to hormone replacement therapy (HRT) are suggested: clonidine and gabapentin. I discuss HRT in the next section, so stick with me here for a bit.

Catapres (clonidine) is a medication seldom used now for the treatment of high blood pressure. If taken by people with normal pressure, it does not lower their blood pressure to any significant degree but does result in some decrease in menopausal symptoms. Unfortunately, there are a number of side effects associated with this drug including dry mouth, dizziness, constipation, and sedation that limit its usefulness.

Neurontin (Gabapentin) is a medication used to control seizures. Like catapres, it does cause some decrease in menopausal symptoms. Studies demonstrate that doses of 900 mg/day, generally given as 300 mg three times a day, are more effective than a placebo. For those with mostly nocturnal symptoms, a dose of 900 mg at night seems to be the most effective. Side effects include headache, dizziness, and disorientation. [13]

I have to admit that few of my patients take either of these medications. This is either because they get home, read the label, and decide not to take it or because, after using it, they find that the benefits don't outweigh the potential risks and side effects. However, if you are not a candidate for hormone replacement therapy and over-the-counter options are not sufficient, you might consider these two medications.

Antidepressants

Some antidepressants, as a side effect, cause a decrease in symptoms. Paxil (paroxetine) at a dose of 7.5 mg daily is the only one currently approved by the FDA for this, but others have been found to have similar effects. Again, if you are not a candidate for hormone replacement therapy and/ or the over-the-counter treatments do not work, you might consider this option.[14]

Hormone Replacement Therapy (HRT)

I consider this category of medications for menopausal symptoms the way I consider Accutane for acne. While many teenagers get zits, most can treat them with over-the-counter topical medication, tetracycline, spironolactone, or birth control pills. For those with severe acne problems, Accutane is the way to go. Why? Because it works. It has risks and side effects, but it works.

---

13. UpToDate, 2020
14. UpToDate, 2020

The same is true for hormone replacement therapy (HRT). While many peri- and postmenopausal women get hot flashes, most can learn to live with them or try lifestyle changes, over-the-counter medications, or the alternative medications discussed previously. For those with symptoms that interfere with life in a meaningful way, they should consider temporary use of HRT. Why? Because it works! It has risks and side effects, but it works.

Before I delve into the various treatment options, I would like to present a brief history of hormone replacement therapy use. Introduced in the 1960s, the original HRT was actually estrogen replacement therapy (ERT) in the form of a medication called Premarin, called such because it was made from pregnant mares' urine. I cannot tell you what compelled respectable scientists to give pregnant mares' urine to women. I won't even hazard a guess. Suffice it to say, it worked. In fact, it was a great success. Menopausal hot flashes and night sweats resolved. Mood swings and vaginal dryness disappeared. Women were very happy. That is, until it was discovered years later that taking continuous, unopposed estrogen over time increased the risk for uterine cancer. Studies found that adding progesterone to counteract the effects of estrogen on the lining of the uterus resulted in a decrease in uterine cancer rates. In fact, the addition of progesterone resulted in levels lower than if the women had taken no medication at all. These findings led to the development of Hormone Replacement Therapy (HRT), rather than simply Estrogen Replacement Therapy (ERT). If you have a uterus, you take both medications; if not, you only take the estrogen. Women were prescribed continuous or cyclic courses depending on whether they wanted to have a period. (Back in those early HRT days, it was considered "feminine" and "young" to have periods. Go figure.)

Not only did this combination work for hot flashes, night sweats, and mood swings, it was also shown to significantly decrease the risk for developing osteoporosis in a time when testing for and treatment of bone loss did not exist. There were no DXA (bone density) scans or bisphosphonates (medications used to treat woman with significant bone loss) at the time. It also slowed the development of cholesterol elevation and heart disease, which typically start at menopause. (Estrogen protects women from these issues prior to menopause. After menopause, their risk for heart disease rapidly climbs to the level of men.) This was in the days before widespread use of statins, a class of drugs used to lower cholesterol levels in the blood, which have proved to be tremendously helpful in reducing cardiovascular disease. In any event, it quickly became fashionable to put all women on HRT at menopause—not only for hot flashes, night sweats, and mood swings, but to preserve the premenopausal elasticity of the vagina and decrease the incidence of painful intercourse. The icing on the cake was that it slowed the development of heart disease and deferred the development of osteoporosis.

But there was a downside. There always is. It was subsequently found that taking HRT for five or more years postmenopausal resulted in a small, but statistically significant, increase in the incidence of breast cancer in those on combined therapy. Also, HRT causes an increased risk for thromboembolic disease, such as strokes and pulmonary embolism. This is most prominently noted upon initiation of treatment but is elevated above the norm throughout use.

Enter the Women's Health Initiative (WHI) in the early 1990s. This study was set up to determine if HRT should be used as a primary preventive measure to decrease heart disease given its beneficial effects on cholesterol. Unfortunately, although a large number of women were enrolled, the cohort in the study did not match the cohort of women who generally took HRT. Some of this came about because the study was designed to exclude women who were symptomatic, i.e. those with hot flashes and night sweats. As a result, the average age of women in the study was 61 rather than 48–50, which was the average age of women entering menopause and being placed on HRT. In addition, there were significantly more smokers in this group than in the population as a whole. In general, those placed on HRT outside of the study tended to be more educated and of higher socioeconomic status with less smokers and better lifestyles. This meant that the average woman in the WHI study was more likely to have preexisting cardiovascular disease. Thus, starting HRT did not result in a decrease in the development of heart disease.

The study did verify that HRT decreased the incidence of osteoporosis and, to a smaller extent, colorectal cancer. There was a small increase in breast cancer in those on combined therapy as mentioned above. However, this was not why the study was stopped. It was for the reasons stated above, it did not demonstrate a decrease in cardiovascular disease. Therefore, HRT could not be recommended for the primary or secondary prevention of heart disease. Unfortunately, that piece got lost in translation, and millions of women immediately stopped taking their HRT, much to their immediate discomfort.

Things have sorted out a bit now, and the general consensus is that HRT is perfectly acceptable for appropriate individuals (e.g., they cannot have recently been diagnosed with breast cancer or have a history of blood clots, pulmonary embolism, or stroke). It is best given at menopause or in the immediate postmenopausal period and should be stopped after five years unless necessary for continued relief of symptoms. Measurement of estrogen and progesterone levels is not necessary during treatment, as the goal is abatement of symptoms, not maintaining a specific level. The good news is that most people don't need HRT for anywhere near that long, so excellent options exist for all.

Estrogen Replacement Therapy (ERT)

Estrogen replacement therapy (ERT) is actually a misnomer. Therapy does not "replace" your estrogen, it simply provides you with enough to treat the symptoms created by the irregularity/loss of estrogen at the time of menopause. Only a small fraction of what you made before menopause is required to treat the symptoms. Measuring the levels in your blood is an unnecessary expense. What you need to treat your symptoms is what you need, no matter what your measured levels are. Average starting doses are generally enough for most women, though many can get along with less, and some will need more. You can start low and work your way up as needed or start higher and wean down. This depends on how severe your symptoms are when you start.

As mentioned previously, the original estrogen replacement was in the form of a drug called Premarin, which was derived from pregnant mares' urine and contains different forms of estrogen that must be metabolized by the liver to estradiol, the form required by the body to enter the cells to do their work. Time and innovation have resulted in the ability to give pure estradiol by mouth. As a result, a debate began concerning natural and unnatural estrogens. For a while, it became fashionable to use estrogen from clover and other plant substances, because this was considered more "natural." In my mind, nothing about clover makes it more natural than pregnant mares' urine. They are both products of nature, although I do agree that the plant-derived versions are more esthetically pleasing than pregnant mares' urine. At the end of the day, no matter the source, it has to be distilled down to estradiol to work. It is available as a pill taken orally, as a patch, as a vaginal suppository or ring, or as topical gel. You can use the more expensive, non-FDA approved creams, salves, and lotions with no assurance that you are getting what you need, or only what you need. I personally vote for the less expensive approved ones. The choice, however, is yours.

The official teaching is that the ERT patches are likely safer, as they bypass the liver and reduce its workload, which can decrease the risk for blood clot formation. If you have liver disease, elevated triglycerides, or gallbladder disease, you might want to consider them. Unfortunately, they cost more than the oral versions, and insurance companies usually require higher co-pays for them.

If you don't have a uterus, ERT is all you need. If you do have a uterus, progesterone needs to be added to protect the lining of the uterus from unopposed estrogen, which can increase the risk for uterine cancer and precancer. As mentioned earlier in the book, if progesterone is given in adequate amounts, not only is the risk for uterine cancer not increased, it is actually less than if you did not use HRT at all.

Progesterone comes in many forms. Provera, the first to be used with Premarin, is a bastardized male hormone tweaked to have progestational properties. In the era of bioequivalency, this medication is often replaced with Prometrium, which is a pure progesterone in tablet form that is taken orally. It is a soporific, which means it makes you sleepy, so best to take it at night. It comes in a peanut oil base, so it should not be taken by those with peanut allergies.

Today, most women choose to take a small daily dose of progesterone rather than the original approach of taking progesterone only on the last 10 to 12 days of the month, which would result in a withdrawal bleed or period. At the time this method was introduced, it was felt that woman would feel younger and more feminine if they bled every month. Fortunately, we know better than that now! Why bleed if you don't have to? You've already paid your dues (not to mention all that you have paid to the feminine product manufacturers and contributed to our ever-growing landfills) by this point in your life.

There are patches that contain estrogen and progesterone if you prefer this method of delivery. (See above for pros and cons.) There are also combination pills containing estrogens and progesterone similar to those in birth control pills but at a much lower level. They are convenient to take and come packaged like birth control pills. Because they are not pure estradiol and progesterone, many opt to take the natural or bioequivalent forms, although data does not exist to show that one is safer than the other over the long term. As far as efficacy goes, both work.

Some women don't tolerate progesterone well because, even at the small levels used in HRT, it can cause unwanted PMS-type symptoms, bloating, and breast discomfort. Women struggling with these side effects can talk with their doctor about periodic withdrawal with progesterone while monitoring the thickness of the lining of their uterus with sonograms. They can also opt to have a progesterone-containing IUD inserted into their uterus, which gives continuous protection with no systemic side effects.

Not to get complicated, but there is a class of drugs containing selective estrogen receptor modulators (SERMs) that, when combined with estrogen, offer protection to the uterus without the side effects of progesterone. They work reasonably well with hot flashes, have less progestational side effects, appear at this time to be "breast neutral," and likely do not increase the risk of blood clots and strokes any more than estrogen already does. More data should be forthcoming.

In contrast to previously held opinions that all women should take estrogen forever, the common approach is to give HRT for no more than five years, as after that point there is a small rise in incidences of breast cancer. Fortunately, most women are through the worst of it in six months to a couple of years. I ask my patients to try each year to cut back on or stop their medication and see what happens. If nothing does, there is no need for you to take a medication you don't need. If bothersome symptoms occur, you have the answer to your question—you need it. Check back next year and see what happens. This cutback can be done cold turkey or slowly decreased over time.

For a minority of women, the vasomotor symptoms, sleep disturbances, muscle and joint aches, or general feeling of well-being consistently return upon cessation of the hormones. Those that don't have contraindications are reminded of the risks and benefits each year and given the opportunity to continue. Current breast cancer is an absolute contraindication, and previous breast cancer is a negotiable contraindication. Risk for thromboembolism is generally low but increases with age, cardiovascular disease, or factors predisposing to cardiovascular disease and family history of blood clotting disorders. Migraine headaches with aura, unlike in premenopausal women on OCPs, are not a contraindication for postmenopausal women interested in HRT.

Many articles tout progesterone as an agent to reduce the incidence of hot flashes; however, most studies do not demonstrate their effectiveness alone (without estrogen) in preventing or treating symptoms. Thus, things like Depo-Provera and vaginal, oral, or topical "gelled" progesterones are not likely to be helpful. The same holds true for testosterone therapy.

Please note that recently, perhaps because of the increasing number of baby boomers who have reached menopausal age, insurance companies have become more aggressive about decreasing the number of women taking

HRT. If you are prescribed these medications, you may well receive a letter from your insurance company, and your doctor will definitely receive communication advising him or her that HRT can cause breast cancer and should be avoided—as if they didn't already know that. Remember, insurance company personnel are not doctors. If you and your physician have, after informed consent, decided that you would best be served by taking these medications, the insurance company cannot legally keep you from taking them. However, they may charge you a ridiculous copay or cover only certain medications that are less costly to them. Try to be flexible. If money is not an issue, which is rarely the case, take what you want. If it is, explore alternatives.

Bioidentical Natural Hormones

Unfortunately, there has been much use and misuse of this term in literature and advertising. As a reaction in the past to the use of pregnant mares' urine in the form of Premarin, which contained many different forms of estrogen, there developed a cottage industry of what are termed bioidentical natural hormones that are chemically similar or structurally identical to estrogen but derived from plant sources such as clover, yams, and soy. These are manipulated in the lab to the form(s) of estrogen generally used by the body. In theory and probably in practice, this makes sense: it's less work for the body to convert these substances to usable forms. However, there is nothing "natural" about the man-made lab process of creating these hormones nor are plants somehow more natural than animals. (If you are vegan, you may want to stick with products derived from plant sources.) At the end of the day, your cells need estradiol to do their work. Initially, the only way a woman could get natural estradiol was from places like the Women's International Pharmacy or from local apothecaries. Unfortunately, the compounding process was not regulated, and women could not be certain of what they were actually getting in terms of dose or purity. That has all changed, and natural hormones are now readily available and regulated by the FDA for safety and efficacy. I personally feel better about taking those than the unregulated ones, but the choice is yours. I must admit that I've had a few patients who felt better served by these alternative medications after trying the FDA-approved ones. Also, be ready to pay a lot more for these compounded products; that payment will likely be out-of-pocket, because many insurance companies will not pick up the cost. In addition, they will likely not cover the costs for blood or salivary estrogen levels, tests that many complementary and alternative medicine (CAM) physicians order to monitor treatment, as the range is wide and dosage will generally be based on efficacy anyway. The dose you end up with is the one that works for you. If you have diabetes or thyroid disease, you are used to measuring levels and adjusting treatment based on the numbers. This does not hold true for HRT

Weight Gain

There are very few women, or men for that matter, over the age of 30 who haven't noticed that they can no longer eat what they want and not gain weight. By 40, many realize that even when they watch what they eat, they gain weight. By 50, the game is over. Simply looking at food seems to put on pounds. This is because the amount of lean muscle a person has begins to decrease at 30 to the tune of 3–8 percent per decade, which can translate to a couple of pounds a year. While that may not sound like much, that means 10–15 pounds over 10 years.

Whether we like it or not, or admit it or not, this decrease in lean muscle is what happens when humans age. We can complain about it, say it's not fair, or refuse to accept it, but, like death and taxes, it is inevitable. Because muscle burns calories much more efficiently than fat, the net effect is what is often referred to as a "slowing of the metabolism" with net gain each year. A 40-year-old sitting still burns less calories than a 30-year-old, a 50-year-old even less, and a 60-year-old less than that. This means that if you eat the same as you did when you were 30 and exercise the same, you will gain weight. You have to eat less and/or exercise more just to maintain. Truth be told, most people exercise less as they age and eat more, so they frequently gain even more than the expected 1-2 pounds a year. In addition, there is a maddening tendency for weight to deposit around the middle during peri- and postmenopause as a result of lower estrogen levels. Even if you don't gain a pound, the distribution of your weight will change as you approach and go through menopause. Those "muffin top" jokes will start to make

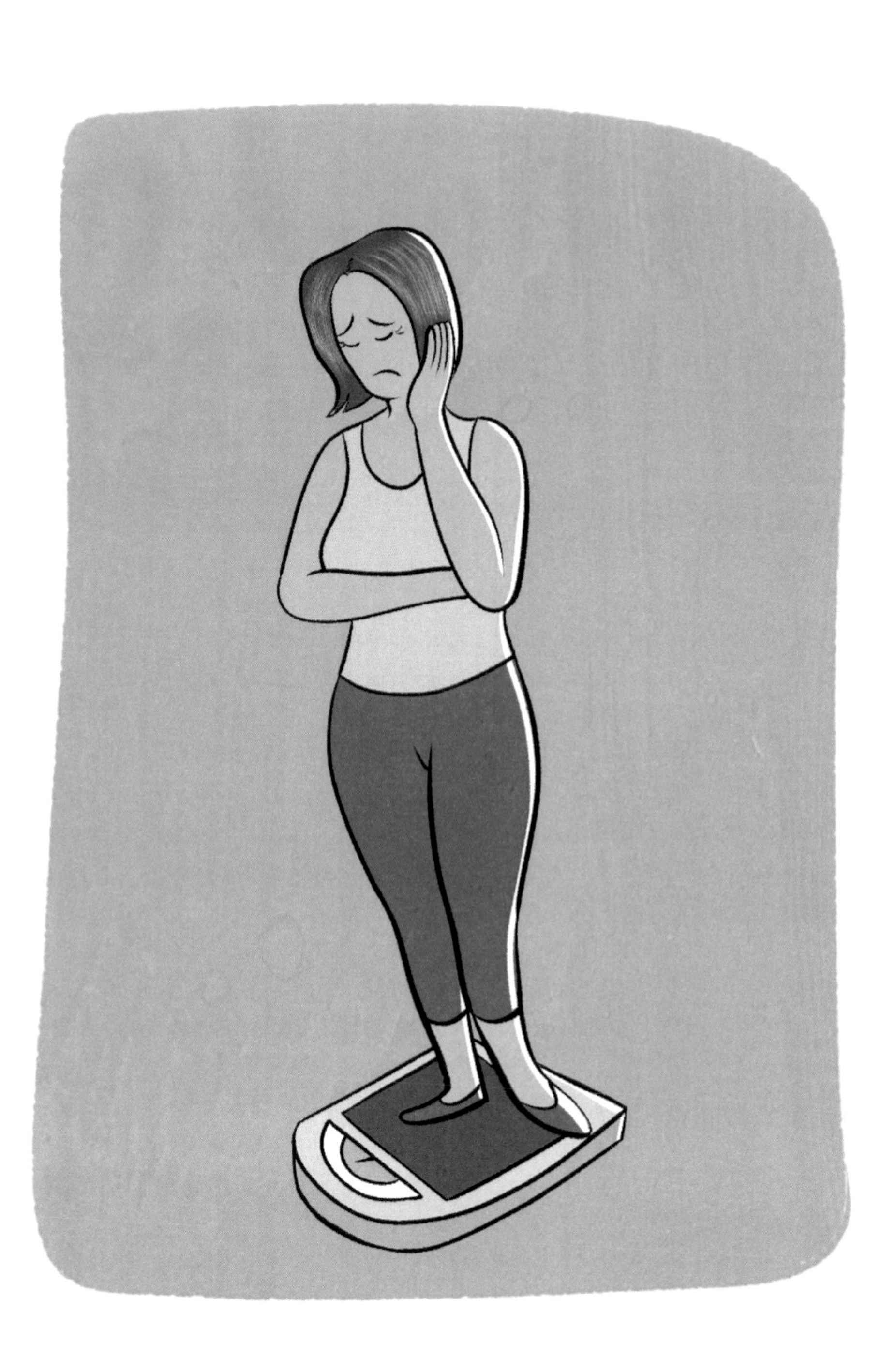

sense to you at this time. You will learn the meaning of Spanx and then Spanx on Spanx. Sadly, at some point after the menopause, nature will win out, and your stomach will look at you and say, "What?!" However, you can stall, or at least minimize, that in the earlier periods before eventually resorting to "mom jeans." If you are at a normal weight and fortunate enough to have the financial capacity, this is a good time to consider a tummy tuck; if that is what you choose to do. However, it is important to recognize that this is not meant as a means to avoid appropriate weight loss. Breast augmentations and/or mastopexies make sense at this time as well before the rest of you starts to sag as much as your pregnancy-associated body parts.

Weight gain is dependent upon a number of variables. Men start off with more lean muscle, so the change is slower. If you were fit in your 20s with lots of lean muscle mass, you start from a higher point and have further to go before you become overweight. Family history plays a role as does lifestyle. If you're lucky, the weight gain may be due to a hormonal cause like hypothyroidism, which does become more common as we age. For the vast majority of women though, the increase is inexorable. Many women make the mistake of trying to decrease their weight to what it was in their 30s. However, because of the reduction of subcutaneous tissue as we age, that weight will look a bit different on you, generally in not a very complimentary way. You could look tired, haggard, or even ill if you attain your numeric goal rather than the one at which you feel comfortable and healthy, no matter the size you wear. Actually, a good trick to play here is to buy more expensive clothes if you are able to do so. I have found from experience that the more money you pay for clothes, the smaller the size on the label; it makes you feel good about spending all of that money even though the amount of material used is the same. A less expensive alternative could be to simply remove the size tag.

What to do? The first thing is to accept reality. If you keep making up excuses for why you gained weight—it's my hormones, it's the pill, it's whatever it is—you won't sign up for the difficult and consistent changes required. If you are not honest with yourself about what you eat and how much you exercise, the same will result.

Diet

I won't even attempt to delve into the literally thousands of diets out there. When patients ask me what I recommend, I have two criteria: is it safe and is it something you will stick to? At the end of the day, they all work by decreasing the total caloric intake. There are no magic foods. If you stick to your diet, and I mean really stick to it, you will lose weight. However, if you chose one that is very restrictive, you may find that the weight comes right back after you finish, because you cannot maintain that lifestyle. Better to choose one that literally changes how you eat and approach food. Please be advised that if you have any health concerns, multiple health problems, and/or dietary restrictions, consult with your medical provider before starting a new diet regimen to help you find and stick to one that is right for you. Below are some of the more popular diets followed by patients in my practice.

Low-Carb Diets: I have to admit that, for years, I was not a believer. I worked out a lot, was in the normal weight category, and I absolutely love rice, pasta, bread, chocolate chip cookies, and ice cream. I had rice or pasta for dinner every night. I would eat a healthy salad for lunch and then add a huge swab of French or Italian bread. I would have a healthy sandwich and follow it with a couple of chocolate chip cookies. Then, it happened… I officially became prediabetic. Time, age, and a family history of diabetes led to my developing an elevated HgbA1c. (HgbA1c is a measure of blood sugar values over time in the blood. Normal is 4.8–5.6. Prediabetes is 5.7–6.4. Diabetes is greater than 6.4.) I did my research and found out how little I really knew about things like glycemic index. Who knew that a bagel and/or a banana for breakfast were not good for those with prediabetes or those following a low carb diet? Now I have nonfat yogurt with blueberries for breakfast and have come to love it. When I do have a bagel, it is scooped out. (I resisted that for a while, but it's really all I need now.) If you can't fill yourself with pasta at dinner, you will take more time to make healthy and delicious veggies and salads. Then, all that is needed is a lean protein source. I used to order salad as a side dish, and now I'm one of those people who will happily eat a large salad for dinner. At first, I felt "not full" but soon realized that feeling was absence of bloating, not the fact that I was actually hungry. In six weeks of adjusting my diet, my HgbA1c dropped from 6.2 to 5.5. In addition, eight pounds magically fell off and have remained off.

Mediterranean Diet: This is a plant-based rather than meat-based diet. Veggies, fruits, nuts, legumes, seeds, fish, and olive oil are promoted. It does include some dairy but limits red meat, processed foods, refined carbohydrates, and unhealthy fats. Recent studies suggest it may promote a more natural and healthier gut biome, which could lead to health benefits beyond those related to obesity and possibly slow the aging process. This diet, like Weight Watchers, has stood the test of time, because it is fact-based, healthy, easy to adhere to, and delicious.

Paleo Diet: I mention this because it is very popular, although I've yet to run into anyone who doesn't make their own substitutions. It does work, because adherents are allowed to eat high-fat, high-protein foods that fill them up and are therefore less likely to cheat. Just a reminder, though: if you look back to the opening paragraph of this book, the average cave man or cave woman did not live long enough to be concerned about high cholesterol, diabetes, or heart disease. Paleo as a jump start? Fine. As a lifestyle, consider switching to a Mediterranean diet, a low-carb diet, or Weight Watchers after the desired weight loss.

Weight Watchers (WW): This oldie but goodie is one that has consistently stood the test of time. It is balanced, healthy, and reasonable in terms of expectations. It is also something that can be followed and/or modified even after the desired weight loss has been achieved. These changes can be made with increased knowledge rather than with prepared meals that cost money, require ordering and delivery, and are, therefore, harder to sustain.

Exercise

If lean muscle burns more calories, work on gaining more lean muscle. Some women tell me they are concerned about looking too much like a jock if they start lifting weights. Believe me, that will not happen overnight or even over months or perhaps years. You don't have to go to a gym where the bodybuilders and want-to-be bodybuilders spend their days working out with the protein drinkers and steroid takers; just add some light strength training activities at least three times a week. Videos, online classes, and home equipment work just as well. Consistency is important here. If you are fortunate enough to have the time and/or money to go to a gym and/or have a personal trainer, you can get assistance with setting up and maintaining a program, but it doesn't have to be complicated or expensive. Small hand weights and/or online videos are widely available. Like the Nike slogan says, "Just Do It."

Aerobic exercise can burn away some of that calorie excess. Regular (at least 3–5 times per week) and consistent aerobic conditioning not only helps with the extra calories, it promotes cardiovascular health, decreases the development of bone loss, helps with mood disorders, and promotes the feeling of general well-being. The more you do, the more you burn. Average calories burned walking for one hour is 100 while runners average 100 calories per mile. In addition, boosts to your metabolism occur when you exercise regularly, and you burn more even when you finish your workout. Aerobic machines give you an average based on your weight. Look at this count when you are done and remember that you can undo that entire hour and 250 calories burned with the "I deserve this now because I exercised" snack or smoothie. This is simple math: calories in vs. calories out.

I've found it is very important to look at regular exercise as an essential and non-negotiable part of your life. You eat every day. You brush your teeth every day. You walk the dog every day. You exercise 3–5 times a week. Period. End of discussion. The question is not if you will exercise this week, it's what days you will exercise this week and what you will do. Yes, life happens. Sometimes there are too many meetings or late nights at work or sick children or illness or ice on the ground or heat waves. If you miss your mark this week, reset it for next week.

Some favorite excuses: it's been too cold (or hot). Well, it gets cold every winter and hot every summer. Wear the appropriate clothing and get moving. (Don't forget to hydrate). Besides, gyms have heat and or air conditioning as does your home or apartment, if you do videos at home. "I don't have the energy to exercise." It takes energy to make energy. Once you get started, you will actually start to feel better. Bottom line is nature does not care what your excuse is. You do not get dispensation because you have a good excuse, which is a reminder of something my father used to say when I was young that infuriated me at the time but makes more sense as time goes on: "That's an excuse, not a reason."

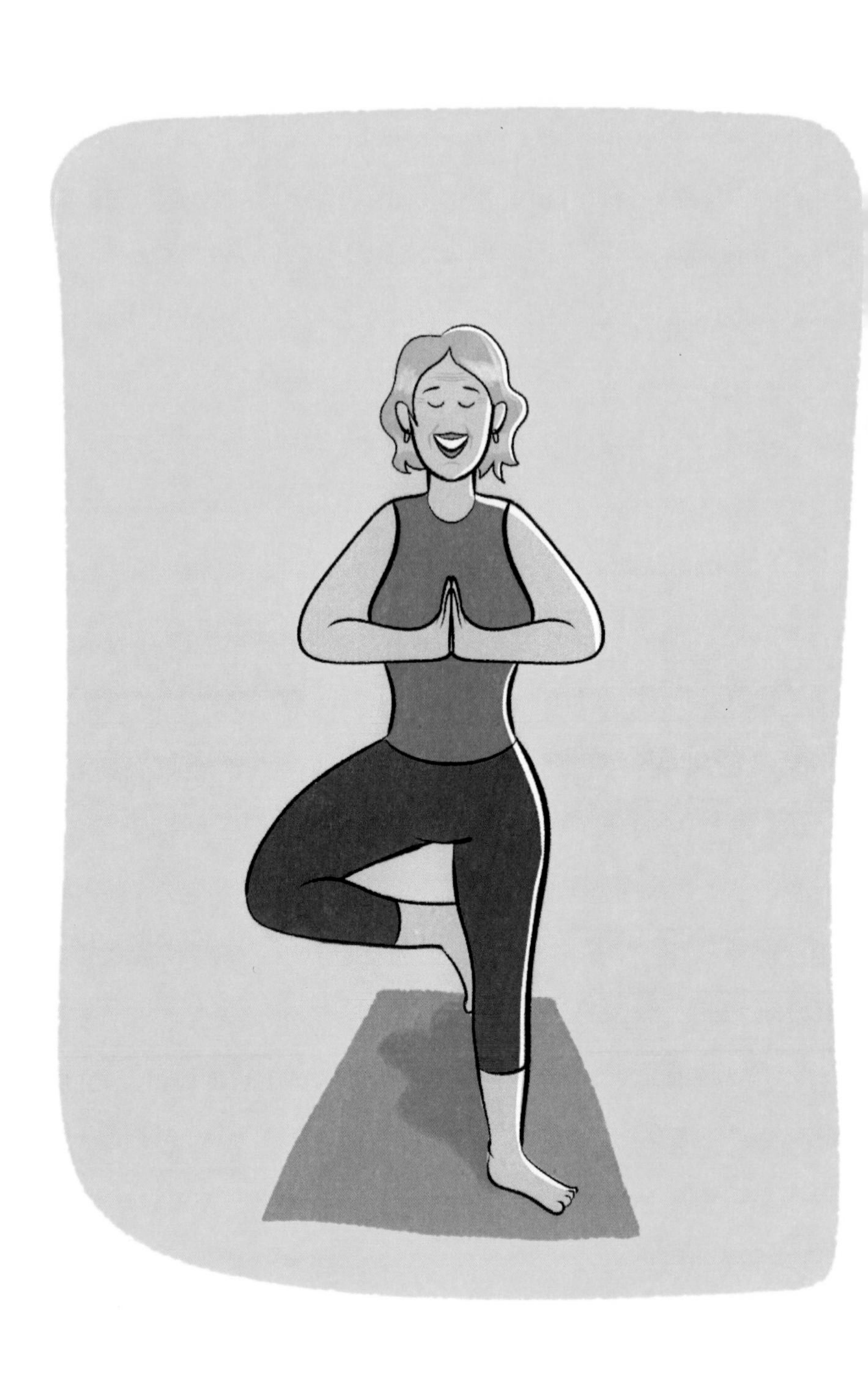

Part Three

Menopause

Technically speaking, a woman is menopausal a year after her last menstrual period. From that point forward, she is technically postmenopausal and no longer produces estrogen in any meaningful amount. This does not happen overnight. Years may pass before there is no measurable estrogen in your system. During this time, your estrogen-dependent organs—your breasts, uterus, vagina, and external genitalia—begin to show changes. Hot flashes and night sweats peak and then, for most, cease.

Alas, there is no more pretending. Welcome to the club! You are now officially old in some people's minds. How did this happen? I still feel like I'm 30! If you do, that's great. One reason may be that we tend to age differently now. Decades ago, women got to their 40s and declared themselves old. They sat down in their chairs. They didn't exercise. They developed muscle aches and pains that compounded their inability to get moving. They ate what they wanted. They got frumpy. Very few of our grandmothers would have considered donning yoga pants, even if they existed, and going to yoga or pilates or barre classes, let alone biking, hiking, kayaking, running, or using a Peloton. They ate what they had always eaten: diets high in carbs, fat, and, therefore, calories. They didn't have the option of shopping at Whole Foods, although they did have the option of Mediterranean diets. They didn't know much about nutrition and often concentrated disproportionately on the carbohydrate portion because carbs are generally cheaper and more plentiful than protein sources and fresh fruits and veggies.

Fortunately, many women approaching menopause are quite different today. They are healthy, vibrant, and young in spirit. This has pushed the new 30 to 40 and sometimes to 50. However, the reality of a body, or any machine for that matter, functioning for that many years begins to add up, and the results become more and more apparent. Does this mean we give up? Absolutely not! But it is the time to take stock and consider how we move forward gracefully, effectively, and safely. We need to sort out which changes are inevitable and which can be prevented, modified, or avoided by lifestyle changes and medication. We cannot change our genetics or how we lived in the past, but we can change how we move forward. Some of this comes by accepting that which cannot be changed and proactively looking for things that can be changed or modified

Vaginal Symptoms

Vulvovaginal atrophy is the medical term used to describe the thinning of vaginal and vulvar tissue immediately prior to and after menopause. These tissues are estrogen-dependent. With the loss of estrogen, they become thinner over time. Biologically, it makes sense. The purpose of these organs is to facilitate intercourse and vaginal delivery. When there are no longer any eggs, as evidenced by a lack of estrogen, the body shuts these organs down. It's sort of like turning off the heat in an area of the house that is not used or having lights go off automatically in a room when there is no movement or escalators that stop running when no one is using them—globally and ecologically responsible. It makes sense when you look at it objectively. Sadly, this can result in painful intercourse, otherwise known as dyspareunia. Many women and their partners want to continue using these organs long past the time they want to reproduce. Hence the problem of painful intercourse.

Many women accept that their hair turns gray or white with aging. They simply color it. They accept that they can't see as well and get bifocals. They accept that they can't run as fast, as far, or can't run at all. They modify their workouts. But, for some reason, they don't accept the vaginal and vulvar changes and bemoan the fact that sex is not like it was when they were in their 30s. If you are honest, you will admit that very little about you post-menopausal is the same as it was in your 30s.

When fully supported, the vaginal and vulvar tissue is thick and turgid, elastic and pliable. Sufficient secretions, or discharge, exist to mitigate against the friction caused by intercourse. After menopause, these properties decrease at variable rates. The vulvar tissue loses fat and the introital area narrows. There is a variable loss in elasticity and vaginal rugae, or series of ridges produced by folding of the vaginal wall. The result is more frequent infections and pain related to intercourse. Your scent may be sharper or "more tart" because the biomes are different due to the lower estrogen level, and the vaginal pH becomes more alkaline. This results from the environmental change, not uncleanliness. Decreased vaginal secretions and elasticity lead to what feels like chapped vaginal tissue, which leads to a sense of friction and tearing during intercourse.

This comes at a time when partners with prostate issues or erectile dysfunction may have more difficulty sustaining an erection. If you are one of those couples who simultaneously are unable to have intercourse, you can either stop or experiment with other pleasurable ways to express your feelings toward each other. Problems arise, however, when one or both of you would like to continue having intercourse. If you are on systemic HRT, you will likely not experience this problem. If not, what to do?

Vaginal Estrogen

There are a number of options. The first is over-the-counter water or silicone-based vaginal lubricants for use with intercourse and moisturizers for use in general but not associated with intercourse. These will be sufficient for many, and there is a plethora of options on the market. Do not be afraid to sample! It's for your own benefit. If those are not enough, there are a number of prescription vaginal estrogens available. The good news is that they work locally, so there are no meaningful amounts in your bloodstream. This is great for those with contraindications to HRT. Most oncologists (cancer specialists) are ok with their use even with women who have or have recovered from breast cancer. These medications encourage the growth of estrogen-dependent cells in the vagina, increase the thickness of the tissue, and allow for more natural lubrication, elasticity, and pliability of the vaginal mucosa.

Treatment comes in the form of creams, tablets, suppositories, and rings that only need to be replaced every three months. Until recently, my discussion with patients was about which form was most acceptable for them. For instance, creams work, but they are messy and can increase the risk for yeast infections. Rings that need replacement only four times a year are very convenient, but many would prefer the twice-weekly tablets (which don't fully dissolve in some women) or suppositories.

Unfortunately, now that a large number of women in this country are postmenopausal and still interested in having intercourse, pharmaceutical companies have raised the price of many of their drugs, and a number of insurance companies have declared vaginal estrogens to be "lifestyle medications," which means they either don't cover them or cover them at a much lower rate. The result is that the average copay in the US for some of these medications has risen from $30 to over $700 in some cases, meaning they are not available for the average woman. (If any of my readers can offer an explanation to me of a marketing plan that would put the price of a medication beyond the reach of most people, I would love to hear from you.) Some women cough up the fee, others find coupons that are occasionally available that cap the copay at $25 or so, which is what I do. Others purchase their medications from Canada. Sadly, most continue to suffer with painful intercourse or give up altogether on the prospect of vaginal sex. Unless things change, I would recommend not setting your mind on a particular form; rather, check to see which one your insurance company will cover at whatever rate they deem to be "usual and customary" and proceed from there.

There are today a number of laser and radio frequency treatments that are touted to treat vulvovaginal symptoms. They are expensive, not covered by insurance, and have variable success rates. To remain symptom-free, you must repeat the treatments on a yearly basis, again at your own expense. You may wish to look into these but know that they are not a panacea.

Postmenopausal Bleeding

Fortunately, most bleeding that occurs in the first year or two after menopause is likely related to that last egg that didn't get asked to dance for a reason. You may suddenly start to feel premenstrual, get cramps, and then have a bleed reminiscent of a period. However, any bleeding that occurs a year or more after menopause needs to be investigated. This is because the risk for uterine cancer or precancer (atypical endometrial hyperplasia) increases with age. If investigation reveals no abnormal findings and you have no further bleeding, that's great. However, if the bleeding persists, you must, as I tell my patients, either bring me a note from God that says you don't have cancer or give me some tissue from your uterus to prove that you don't have abnormal cells. That tissue from your uterus comes in the form of an endometrial biopsy (EMB). While uncomfortable, I have had one; it is tolerable. I have never understood why some physicians tell their patients it will feel like a pinch. It's not a pinch! It hurts, and it hurts more if you are postmenopausal, especially if you have not had any vaginal deliveries to stretch open your cervix. I find it better to advise my patients of the potential discomfort than to have them surprised, shocked, or upset with me for being untruthful. I offer those patients with a low pain threshold or high anxiety levels ways to reduce the discomfort. That along with, or perhaps instead of, a sonogram to evaluate the thickness of the lining of your uterus, or endometrial stripe, can rule out significant abnormality in most cases. Stripes less than 5 mm are infrequently associated with uterine cancer or precancer. In general, uterine cancer is user-friendly in that it tends to raise its hand early and identify itself with unexpected bleeding. If diagnosed early, a hysterectomy will be necessary. No chemo or radiation is required. If ignored, it becomes as unfriendly as any cancer that progresses to advanced stages.

Vaginal atrophy is a less common cause of postmenopausal bleeding. After years without estrogen support, the vaginal tissue in some women becomes so thin and atrophic (shrinkage or thinning of muscle or nerve tissue) that bleeding results from intercourse or even in its absence. The bleeding is painless and generally light. After ruling out other causes, treatment with vaginal estrogen should result in relief.

Osteoporosis

Until menopause, most women, except those with anorexia or those on steroids for a number of medical illnesses, are protected from this devastating condition of low bone mass or density with resultant deterioration and fragility, leading to an increase risk for fracture with minor trauma. Estrogen supports bone growth and positively affects the delicate balance between loss and growth. Prior to menopause, there is typically a regular net gain in bone mineral density, although this gain decreases yearly after about 30. After menopause, the net loss begins to increase. Depending on family history, ethnicity and lifestyle, you may soon find yourself developing osteopenia, a condition where bone loss or density is lower than considered healthy, but not yet to the point where fractures occur with minor trauma as in osteoporosis. You are most at risk if you are a thin, white female who smokes, drinks, and has a strong family history. The bone density you have when you reach menopause is determined by genetics and lifestyle. Whatever you have at that time, you will begin to see a yearly loss. The rate of loss and the peak density at menopause determine when or if you will be at risk for osteoporosis development in later years.

The good news is that we can measure bone density through DXA scans. The absolute numbers are compared with healthy premenopausal women not at risk for fracture. Over time, as you lose bone, you may find that your bone density goes below a certain level (-1.5) and you are diagnosed with osteopenia. At this point, you should take heed but not worry. You have time to build more bone. Weight-bearing exercise and adequate calcium and vitamin D consumption along with smoking cessation can help you maintain and/or rebuild your bone density. Regular (3–5 times a week) weight-bearing exercises like walking and strength training challenge your bones to rebuild. Swimming, while a great exercise in general, does not challenge your bones in the same way because the body weight is held up by the water.

Adequate calcium, aka 1,000-1,200 mg per day is required. This should be obtained through diet as much as possible. Dairy products and calcium-fortified nondairy products, such as almond or soymilk, are the sources with the largest amount of calcium per serving. While green leafy vegetables are high in calcium for vegetables, large amounts are required to reach the daily allowance. One cup of broccoli provides only 100 mg of calcium. Unfortunately, humans lack the enzymes necessary to release the calcium in spinach. If supplements are required, please note that the body can only absorb 500 – 600 mg of calcium at a time, so do not take your entire daily amount at one sitting because half of it will not be absorbed. Vitamin D helps absorb calcium which, along with protein, is needed to build bone. If you have not recently done so, please have your level checked. There is no need to add more vitamin D to your diet if your levels are normal.

If your density falls below -2.5, you have osteoporosis and are at an increased risk of fracture with minor trauma. Morbidity and mortality increase significantly once this occurs. Fractured hips are associated with long-term stays in medical facilities, decreased mobility, and overall increased mortality. There are a number of medications that help increase bone density like alendronate (Fosamax), ibandronate (Boniva), and denosumab (Prolia). They are often expensive and have side effects but prove well worth it as compared to the alternative of being on a walker, disabled, or dying early.

A Guide to Calcium-Rich Foods

We all know that milk is a great source of calcium, but you may be surprised by all the different foods you can work into your diet to reach your daily recommended amount of calcium. Use the guide below to get ideas of additional calcium-rich foods to add to your weekly shopping list.

Produce	**Serving Size**	**Estimated Calcium***
Collard greens, cooked	1 cup	266 mg
Broccoli rabe, cooked	1 cup	100 mg
Kale, cooked	1 cup	179 mg
Soybeans, cooked	1 cup	175 mg
Bok Choy, cooked	1 cup	160 mg
Figs, dried	2 figs	65 mg
Broccoli, fresh, cooked	1 cup	60 mg
Oranges	1 whole	55 mg
Seafood	**Serving Size**	**Estimated Calcium***
Sardines, canned with bones	3 oz	325 mg
Salmon, canned with bones	3 oz	180 mg
Shrimp, canned	3 oz	125 mg
Dairy	**Serving Size**	**Estimated Calcium***
Ricotta, part-skim	4 oz	335 mg
Yogurt, plain, low-fat	6 oz	310 mg

Milk, skim, low-fat, whole	8 oz	300 mg
Yogurt with fruit, low-fat	6 oz	260 mg
Mozzarella, part-skim	1 oz	210 mg
Cheddar	1 oz	205 mg
Yogurt, Greek	6 oz	200 mg
American Chees	1 oz	195 mg
Feta Cheese	4 oz	140 mg
Cottage Cheese, 2%	4 oz	105 mg
Frozen yogurt, vanilla	8 oz	105 mg
Ice Cream, vanilla	8 oz	85 mg
Parmesan	1 tbsp	55 mg
Fortified Food	**Serving Size**	**Estimated Calcium***
Almond milk, rice milk or soy milk, fortified	8 oz	300 mg
Orange juice and other fruit juices, fortified	8 oz	300 mg
Tofu, prepared with calcium	4 oz	205 mg
Waffle, frozen, fortified	2 pieces	200 mg
Oatmeal, fortified	1 packet	140 mg
English muffin, fortified	1 muffin	100 mg
Cereal, fortified	8 oz	100-1,000 mg

Other	Serving Size	Estimated Calcium*
Mac & cheese, frozen	1 package	325 mg
Pizza, cheese, frozen	1 serving	115 mg
Pudding, chocolate, prepared with 2% milk	4 oz	160 mg
Beans, baked, canned	4 oz	160 mg

**The calcium content listed for most foods is estimated and can vary due to multiple factors. Check the food label to determine how much calcium is in a particular product.*[15]

Prevention is the key here. I liken it to your 401(k). The more money you put in while you are young, the more you have when you need to withdraw. As you age, exercises like tai chi and yoga become more important as they increase balance and the awareness of yourself in space. This decreases the risk of falling. My most poignant experience in this regard was a winter day when I was returning to my car after working out with my trainer, Tony, who is also a physical therapist. Throughout every session, Tony reminded me to "tighten the core." On that particular winter day, I returned to my car after working out and noticed a huge wad of compacted ice and snow on the front tire. I kicked it off but didn't realize I was standing on a thin sheet of ice. I started to fall backwards and could, in my mind, see the trajectory of a protractor predicting the ultimate result of the back of my head hitting the concrete. It was then that I could hear Tony telling me to "tighten the core!" I immediately contracted my abs and stopped the backward fall. I will love him forever for saving me that day.

Falls can be a game changer, so it is essential to take the time to fall-proof your house sooner rather than later. Remove all throw rugs and/or fasten them down. Remove all clutter, especially before you go to bed. Install grab bars as indicated. Use night lights to allow you to see on those inevitable nightly trips to the bathroom; since your bladder is no longer flush with

15. National Osteoporosis Foundation

estrogen, you'll need to urinate more frequently. Talk with your primary care doctor about medications that might dull your senses and increase your risk for falls.

Medications

Bisphosphonates became available in the 1980s and did much to decrease the devastating consequences of bone loss over time. These medications affect the balance between osteoclasts, which break down bone, and osteoblasts, which build up bone. Prior to menopause, more bone is built than broken down. After menopause, there is a reverse in this process with more bone being broken down than built up. The bisphosphonates like Fosamax and Boniva allow for a net gain in bone density. When first available, they were recommended for osteopenia (bone loss) and osteoporosis (bone loss associated with increased risk for fracture.) Many women were placed on this drug. Over time, it became clear that the risk-benefit ratio supported the use of these drugs for those with osteoporosis but not for osteopenia because of side effects like transverse femoral fractures which were rare prior to widespread use of these drugs. Truth be told, these fractures are not associated with significant disability but can be avoided with appropriate screening. If your risk for osteoporosis is low, then medication is not needed. If your risk is high, better to get a transverse fracture that heals than a hip fracture that results in permanent disability.

Prolia and Reclast are the next steps if the bisphosphonates do not work or have been "timed out" after five years of treatment. They offer continued protection and should be explored if you remain at risk. Insurance usually requires an adequate trial of bisphosphonates prior to their use, as they are much more expensive. Some insurance companies actively discourage the use of these medications, likely because they are expensive. In my mother's case, every time she was given a refill for her Fosamax, the insurance company first insisted she try calcium and vitamin D despite the fact that she had documented osteoporosis and an osteoporosis-related fracture.

Breast Cancer

Sadly, the incidence of breast cancer increases with age. The longer a woman has breasts, the higher her risk for getting breast cancer. However, older women diagnosed with breast cancer tend to have less aggressive cases than those in younger or premenopausal women, who tend to have genetic predispositions to early and more aggressive cancers. Screening for breast cancer genes (BrCa) is important in families with this history. Cancer is easier to diagnose mammographically in postmenopausal women due to their thinner tissue from lack of estrogen. There is no consensus yet in this country as to what age women should stop regular mammogram screenings, as a lot depends on the life expectancy of each woman getting the screens and her medical history. Despite the small increased risk for women taking hormone replacement therapy, most women who get breast cancer never took hormone replacement; if you need to use it, you should not be unnecessarily concerned.

Gynecologists now encourage breast self-awareness rather than breast self-exams. Self-exams have the connotation of being tests that can be failed, whereas self-awareness means that each woman is an expert on what her breasts normally feel like. If an irregularity is noted, all they have to do is bring their breast and a finger to point to the irregularity. Her provider can take it from there. You should also know that many women with a history of, or increased risk for, breast cancer take tamoxifen (a drug called an "aromatase inhibitor" that has pro- and anti-estrogen like properties) to decrease their risk for recurrence or development of breast cancer. This drug can cause and/or aggravate menopausal symptoms.

Decreased Libido

One of my older male colleagues once said to me, "Women need a reason to have sex. Men need a place." While, in general, it is true that there is a strong emotional component to sex for many, if not most, women, time and waning hormones can wreak havoc with the desire and/or ability for men and women to have satisfactory sexual relations. When obtaining a history from my patients at their annual, I generally ask my premenopausal patients if they have any pain or problems with intercourse. At and after menopause, I ask first if they are sexually active. This is because the frequency of intercourse decreases significantly as women age. Some of this may be due to the fact that they have been with the same partner for decades, which in and of itself will likely result in decreased frequency (but that is a subject for a different book). However, libido does decrease with time and age. A good amount can be attributed to the fact that sex begins to hurt when estrogen levels wane. The previous segments on vaginal symptoms and vaginal estrogen address options for dealing with that.

For others, the decrease happens despite appropriate vaginal lubrication and pliability. Some may be related to their partner's issues with prostate and erectile dysfunction, and some may be related to chronic disease, depression, or the use of certain medications by the woman or her partner. For example, selective serotonin reuptake inhibitors, (SSRIs) are a widely used class of antidepressants that increase levels of a "feel-good" chemical substance in the brain called serotonin. They are particularly well known for their association with decreased libido and/or inability to achieve orgasm. However, for a growing number of aging women, interest in sex wanes without any of the above. This decrease in libido, or hypoactive sexual desire disorder, is greatest in women aged 40–60 or earlier if they have undergone surgical menopause.[16]

Some may be related to unrealistic expectations of being a "sex kitten" with multiple orgasms that just does not happen in most cases as we age. Some may be related to the goal-oriented society we live in where the goal—orgasm—becomes more important than the interaction. Things change with time, and body image affects intimacy. Remember that your partner likely doesn't look exactly the same as they did when you first met. Orgasm may be delayed or not occur at all, but that does not negate the pleasurable and intimate feelings that intercourse/sexual intimacy can bring. Adjustment may be required. Please be advised that if your libido was low before menopause, it will not likely improve afterwards. Realistic expectations are needed here. There are differences between avoidance, dislike, and just not

16. Practice Bulletin, 2019

on the agenda. More importantly, if it is ok with you and ok with your partner not to have vaginal intercourse, there is really no reason to rock that boat. Communicate in loving ways that augment and stabilize your relationship rather than chasing dreams of youth that may no longer apply. You've been together this long for a reason in most cases. Remember that there are therapists who specialize in female sexual dysfunction and pelvic floor physical therapy. Consider availing yourself of one of these professionals if the issue is affecting your relationship and/or your feelings of self-worth.

As a note, you may come across information about Viagra-type equivalents for women touted as medications to increase libido. You should know that Viagra came about by accident. It was being used in a trial for the treatment of elevated blood pressure in men in Scotland. The study found no significant benefit in decreasing blood pressure; however, at the end of the trial, participants were reluctant to return their remaining pills. It turns out that their use resulted in an increase in the frequency, strength, and duration of erections. The rest is history. This medication works by increasing blood flow to the penis, which allows for a functional erection. It has nothing to do with libido, which is why the equivalents in women have not been successful. Women are unlike men in so, so many ways!

Testosterone Therapy

Male hormone levels in women decrease in the pre and perimenopausal periods and stabilize at this new low with the cessation of menses. While the use of testosterone has been shown in a number of studies to increase desire and activity, not all of them do, and many of the trials involved small numbers of women. There is much research going on in this area today, but we are in the infancy stages of using male hormones for decreased sexual desire. Some gynecologists and/or sexual medicine specialists have developed a great deal of interest and experience in this area and keep abreast of the latest research. If this is something you wish to look into, ask your provider to refer you to one. Please note that the use of male hormones may increase the risk for male-related complications, such as elevated cholesterol, diabetes, heart disease, acne, unwanted hair growth, and masculinization of the female genitalia. There have also been sporadic reports of increased risk for breast cancer with its use. Choose your poison here—it is not a panacea.

Weight Gain

Part Two contains a thorough discussion about this "malady." To that I would like to add the following additional observations.

By 50, many women are understandably frustrated by their inability to maintain or lose weight. Please understand that, even though the distribution of weight changes after menopause with an unremitting tendency to weight around the middle, our bodies change as well with less subcutaneous fat. If, in fact, we did weigh what we did in our 30s, we would look tired, drawn, and gaunt. A little extra weight at this time can be just fine. That is, if you were not overweight to begin with. What is overweight? A body mass index (BMI) of 25 or more is considered overweight, whereas obese is a BMI of 30 or more, and morbid obesity is a BMI over 40. Women with a BMI of less than 25 may be distressed that they have gained weight, but they are still healthy. Your ego may be hurt, and you may have to buy new clothes, but your health will likely not be impacted. BMIs over 30 bring increased risk for high cholesterol, high blood pressure, and diabetes, all of which increase the risk of cardiovascular disease and certain cancers.

At their annuals, many of my older patients bemoan their inability to lose weight while claiming they are doing everything right. Truth be told, after discussion, women often provide additional feedback that helps to explain some of the problem. For instance, while they may be eating all of the right things, they also frequently eat the wrong things. Their "healthy" salads are often smothered with caloric dressing and all of the other add ons like breadcrumbs and the like. May as well just have that cookie with a less caloric salad. Working women frequently complain they don't have time to cook. Last I checked, yogurt, fruit and nuts, and many veggies don't require any preparation. As for exercising, I agree that most do not have much energy when they come home, but once you start exercising, you get more energy You just have to get started. "I used to exercise regularly" is a favorite excuse as if past behavior will cover their current inactivity.

That's like saying, "I used to pay my rent, but I no longer do." If you stop exercising, you will gain weight. They say they use aerobics machines, but upon further questioning, the use is sporadic and/or they do it for 15–20 minutes at a pace that would burn about 75–100 calories in an hour if they actually did it that long. When I'm at the gym, I see 30-year-olds running on the treadmill for an hour and 50-year-olds walking for 15–20 minutes. The kicker is that they don't sweat while performing the exercises and frequently reward themselves with an extra helping at dinner. For the life of me, I don't understand why people watch the Food Network while exercising. That can only lead to their undoing when they finish. By the way, "glistening" may be proper and ladylike, but only drenching sweat will do the trick to burn substantial calories.

Bottom line is that many have convinced themselves they are doing the best they can. Maybe they are. If so, they must resign themselves to continued weight gain. If not, they need to step it up. Sound harsh? I didn't make the rules—I am telling you what nature has decided they are. Accept and do what is required and maintain, or don't accept, don't do what is required, and continue to gain or not lose weight. It's like saying you want $100,000 in your 401(k) but don't want to take a larger percentage out of your salary or work more. You will not reach your goal, which means you will have to adjust your budget. Nature absolutely does not care. We do not get a vote here. Every day you make a choice between comfort and overweight and discomfort and desired weight. Clearly, for the majority, the choice is for the former. Okay. So that's your choice. Own it and move on.

At this point, those on HRT tend to blame it for their weight gain. Those not on HRT blame that for weight gain. Look at your spouse or the other men in your life. They too are gaining weight, albeit more slowly, because they have more calorie-burning lean muscle than most women. The only thing you can legitimately blame lack of estrogen for is the maddening placement of much of that extra weight around the middle, something I have formally decided to accept—not without a tremendous fight, I might add.

Emotional Symptoms

Part Two contains a more thorough discussion about this topic. To that I would like to add that many nonhormonal changes occur at this time in life. If you had children, depending on how old you were when you had your babies, your children may now be in college, graduate school, or on their own. This is a significant life event that requires adjustments to how you perceive yourself and your role in life. Gone are the days when women in their 40s and 50s could expect grandchildren to take the place of their grown children. Most now are preparing for a least a decade or longer before they will be grandparents. Many women now have careers and may have reached the pinnacle of those careers at this point in their life. Those who aren't satisfied with where they have landed may be looking to recreate themselves or learn new skills. They have often been married to the same person for over half of their lives and now have time to examine that relationship and make decisions. Adding symptoms like hot flashes, night sweats, and emotional lability to that equation makes it more challenging. Time to sort things out and re-emerge as the person you want to be.

Redistributed Hair

Many women note with distress a loss of hair in the peri and postmenopausal period and/or hair in places they didn't have it before, such as on their upper lip and/or chin. This is due to a decrease in estrogen while testosterone levels remain relatively the same, resulting in an overall dominance of male hormone. Low thyroid or elevated testosterone levels can result in hair loss but are generally associated with other clinical signs and symptoms. For most women, testing for these abnormalities is likely to be normal, and you will have to live with it. Family history of hair loss does not help here. There are few things more distressing than having more hair on your chin than on your scalp. Medications such as Rogaine as well as shaving, threading, waxing, and laser hair removal remain options. If you plan to do it yourself with tweezers, please remember that a magnified mirror will likely be required after you get to this stage. I personally choose the young eyes of a threader to accomplish my goals. The good news is that as hair is disappearing from your head it is also becoming sparser under your arms and in the pubic area, so you can spend less time removing/taming those hairs.

Cognitive Changes a.k.a. Brain Fog

Increased cognitive changes are a frequent complaint of peri and post-menopausal women. A comic that comes to mind illustrates someone in a room with smoke billowing through the door and a fire extinguisher on the wall; the caption read: "I came in here for a reason, I hate it when I forget things." At age 50, word-finding and name recall is not an uncommon complaint, but many women fast-forward from forgetting someone's name to fearing they have Alzheimer's disease. When we need bifocals to see better, we don't automatically assume that we will be blind soon. When our hair begins to thin, we don't automatically assume that we will be bald tomorrow. Yet, when we forget someone's name, we immediately assume that we will have Alzheimer's tomorrow and be placed in a memory care unit. The art of the game is to try to understand which changes are normal and which are pathologic. Sadly, there are no foolproof ways to do that yet. Data suggests that there may be a fast-forwarding of cognitive changes in menopause that eventually equilibrates, but we can only wait for more research at this point.

Other Menopausal/Aging Concerns

Muscular/Joint Aches and Pains

There are numerous causes of muscle and joint aches and pains in women of all ages. I will not even pretend to cover this area in any sort of completeness. Suffice it to say that many women (and men as well) note an increase in these symptoms as they age, but not necessarily because they are related to menopause. Part of aging involves wear and tear on the joints. We push our bodies, perhaps too much at times, with activities like tennis, running, biking, and high-intensity interval training (HIIT); this can lead to replacement surgeries later in life. We women tend to aggravate that with "cute shoes." I, heretofore, had been quite guilty of that. Discomfort was, in my mind, well worth the cost of looking good. However, searing hip and/or knee pain was not. As a result of a consultation with an orthopedic surgeon, I am now building a wardrobe of "cute" flats, tightening my core with pilates, and happily and gratefully experiencing little to no pain.

For those with an increase in muscular and/or joint pain symptoms not related to their "cute shoes," there are indeed a number of women who fare better with HRT after menopause. My belief is that women should be given that option and monitored. There are also a good number who note an improvement in their symptoms with nonsteroidal anti-inflammatory drugs (NSAIDs) or change/elimination of certain exercise regimens and/or the additions of new ones, especially those that concentrate on core strengthening. Clearly, there is not one answer to the question. Literally, one size fits none. Keep it in mind though, and if muscular and/or joint pain is an issue for you, please discuss this with your provider.

Migraine Headaches

Many women note a significant improvement or lessening in the frequency of their migraine headaches at and after menopause. The relationship between migraines and hormones makes sense, since the frequency of migraines is significantly higher in premenopausal women than men. Please note that while migraines with aura are a contraindication to OCP use, they are not a contraindication to HRT use.

Dry and Crepe Skin

While scaly skin is revered in the reptilian world, most humans would rather not be able to relate so well to alligators. Many menopausal women wonder if estrogen therapy will keep them looking young and/or reverse the changes that have already begun. In my mind, this is sort of like the fact that most basketball players are tall, but not all tall people are basketball players. Most women who have estrogen are young. Therefore, their skin is young as are all parts of their body. As we age, there is a decrease in collagen in the skin and a decrease in the amount of fat beneath the skin (the only place we would actually want any more fat on our bodies at this time). This along with decreased elasticity leads to drooping or sagging of the skin. Dryness increases, and there is more itching and irritation. (This can be especially aggravating in vulvar tissue, and external estrogen can help here.) The repair process is slowed, and recovery and replacement of damaged skin is hindered. These changes happen with or without estrogen, although for some, the additional fluid retention noted while on HRT can cause a plumping effect on the face, making it appear a bit younger. Besides age, family history and photoaging due to sun exposure are generally the biggest determinants of how your skin looks. You certainly cannot choose your genetics, but you can definitely avoid sun exposure and use liberal amounts of protection when you do go out. There are retinoid creams, injections, surgeries, and various resurfacing procedures with lasers or chemicals that may be beneficial here. Alas, estrogen is not a panacea for normal aging.

Women have been known to go to great lengths and spend incredible amounts of money to preserve their youthful appearance. Many insurance companies do not cover these alternative medical treatments and supplements. Between the consultation appointments, possible lab work, supplements, procedures, and other hormonal treatments, one could easily spend several thousand out-of-pocket dollars annually on these treatments. If you have the discretionary income and see or feel real benefit from these treatments, go for it.

In summary, based on the above information, the following are indications for consideration of HRT use in perimenopausal and postmenopausal women:

- Vasomotor Symptoms a.k.a. Hot Flashes: These are the most common reasons for taking HRT and most likely to be resolved or at least lessened by HRT.
- Sleep Disturbances: If related to menopause, significant improvement in these symptoms can be obtained with HRT. Unfortunately, in today's nonstop world, many people are plagued by insomnia—menopausal or not. HRT is not a

panacea for all causes, but it can help those individuals with sleep loss secondary to estrogen decrease or irregularities.

- Mood Swings and/or Depression: I once had a patient make an appointment to discuss starting HRT. She was perimenopausal and having some hot flashes, but they were minor. Her biggest concern was her mood swings, irritability, sadness, and depression. In going over what was happening in her life, it turns out she had just left her husband who had been unfaithful, her young daughter had run off with a guy in a rock band who used lots of drugs, her family business was about to declare bankruptcy, her mother had cancer, and the beloved family dog had just died. Clearly her symptoms were justified, but not because she was perimenopausal. At her insistence, I prescribed HRT. In follow-up, she felt that, while her life was still in shambles, her ability to tolerate her situation was much improved. Not a panacea, but a great help. Lesson learned.

- Bone Loss: Most women with significant bone loss are best served by medications specifically designed to alter the balance between the cells that break bone down and those that build it up. However, if you have significant menopausal symptoms AND are beginning to lose bone, ERT/HRT may be the best option for you.

- Stress Urinary Incontinence: Both vaginal and systemic estrogen can be helpful for women with this concern.

- Muscular/Joint Aches and Pains: We don't know why this occurs, but it does. Those whose lives are negatively impacted by the limitations of muscular and/or joint aches and pains often continue therapy for years.

Aging vs. Menopausal Changes

	Menopause	Aging	Both
Cognitive Changes	?	X	
Skin Changes		X	
Hair Loss			X
Bone Loss			X
Decreased Libido			X
Weight Gain		X	
Weight Distribution	X		
Muscular / Joint Aches and Pains			X
Stress Urinary Incontinence			X

Conclusion

The majority of women reading this book have the privilege of living in a first-world country. In addition, many have access to top-of-the-line medical care and the wherewithal to adopt positive lifestyles. All have the advantage of living in the 21st century. To that end, you can reasonably expect to live a long and productive life, especially if you have been blessed with good genetics and live a healthy lifestyle. That's the good news. The bad news is that, whether we like or accept it or not, we will all age. With that comes a number of unwelcome but inevitable changes. The challenge to all is to have the wisdom to learn what we can to optimize what time we have left and the grace to accept what we can and cannot change. Life is a precious gift. Enjoy and, in the words of Dr. Spock from *Star Trek*, "live long and prosper."

Author's Notes

Much has changed since I started my career in the 1980s and when I personally started to go through my menopausal journey, which, sadly, still continues to this day! It is becoming much more commonplace and accepted today to discuss issues and symptoms related to this stage of life. It is no longer viewed as a stigma. On the contrary, it has become a great marketing opportunity for products and services to baby boomers and Gen-Xers. Good for us!

In general, the more knowledge one has, the better—to a point, anyway. In doing research for this book and perusing the infamous "journal of the internet," I came across some remarkably scary misinformation based on lack of understanding of basic science, purposeful misrepresentation of facts in order to sell products, or simply a mistrust of medical personnel as if we had pledged some kind of oath to do harm rather than the oath of Hippocrates to "…follow that system of regimen which, according to my ability and judgment, I consider for the benefit of my patients, and abstain from whatever is deleterious and mischievous.[17] I have a cup on my desk that says, "Please do not confuse your Google research for my medical degree." Many today tend to do just that and assume they know as much, if not more, than their physicians after their foray into the "journal of the internet." Do your research, please. Ask all of the questions you need to ask

17. Encyclopedia Britannica, 2020

and choose a doctor you feel comfortable with whose philosophies match yours to take you through your journey.

Thank you for purchasing my book. I hope it has provided you with the insights and information you were seeking and that it will serve as an ongoing resource for you during your menopausal journey.

I would welcome your feedback on the book and encourage you to visit and bookmark my website at https://askdrheatherjohnson.com and follow me on Facebook (@askdrheatherjohnson), Instagram (@askdrheatherjohnson), and Twitter (@askdrjohnson) for additional information as well as more of my Dr. J's Pearls.

Glossary

American College of Obstetricians and Gynecologists (ACOG): a professional association of physicians specializing in obstetrics and gynecology in the United States

Adenomyosis: Growth of cells that normally line the uterine cavity in the muscular layers of the uterus causing uterine enlargement, cramps and/or excessive bleeding

Anorexia: A psychological disorder that results in excessive weight loss due to refusal to eat.

Anti-Müllerian Hormone (AMH): A hormone made in reproductive tissues

Antidepressant: A medication used to treat depression

Atresia: Degeneration of tissue

Atypical Endometrial Hyperplasia: Enlargement or overproduction of uterine lining cells

Bioequivalent: Biological agents that are the same

Bisphosphonates: Medications used to treat bone loss

Boniva: A medication used to treat bone loss

BrCa testing: Blood test for genes that predispose to breast cancer

Chronic Fatigue Syndrome: A disorder characterized by extreme fatigue and pain with, as yet, an unknown cause

Complementary and Alternative Medicine (CAM): health care approaches that are not typically part of conventional / traditional Western medical care (i.e., Acupuncture, Reflexology, yoga and other mind-body therapy, natural herbal products, etc.)

Climacteric: A time in life where female estrogen levels decline. It ends at menopause.

Connective Tissue Disease: An autoimmune disorder where your immune system attacks healthy cells

Depo-Provera: A progesterone drug used for birth control that is given as an injection every three months

DXA Scan: An x-ray test used to measure the density of bone

Donor Egg: An egg donated from one individual to allow pregnancy in another

Dyspareunia: Pain with intercourse

Ectopic Pregnancy: Pregnancy occurring outside the uterine cavity

Endometrium: Cells lining the uterine cavity

Endometrial Ablation: A procedure to remove a thin layer of tissue (endometrium) that lines the uterus to stop or reduce heavy menstrual bleeding

Endometrial Biopsy (EMB): Sampling of cells from the lining, endometrium, of the uterus

Endometrial Polyp: Fleshy growth of tissue in the uterus made of the cells that normally line the uterine cavity

Endometrial Stripe: A measure of the thickness of the lining of the uterine cavity

Endometriosis: The growth of uterine lining cells outside of the uterine cavity onto other pelvic organs

Estradiol: A female hormone

Estrogen: A female hormone

Estrogen Replacement Therapy (ERT): Female hormone used to replace natural hormones after the menopause

Fallopian Tube: One of two structures that extend from the top of the uterus and end atop the ovaries to allow transport of eggs

Fibroids: Benign muscular and stromal tissue growths in the wall of the uterus

Fibromyalgia: A medical condition associated with widespread musculoskeletal pain

Fimbria: The terminal end of the fallopian tubes that extend over the ovaries

Fertility Preservation: Freezing of a woman's eggs at a younger age to extend her reproductive capacity

Follicle Stimulating Hormone (FSH): A hormone secreted by the pituitary gland that includes the growth of eggs in the ovary

Fosamax: A medication used to treat loss of bone associated with osteoporosis

Gardasil 9 (Human Papillomavirus 9-Vaccine): A vaccine for use in the prevention of certain strains of cancers caused by HPV (Types 6, 11, 16, 18, 31, 33, 45, 52, and 58)

HgbA1C (Hemoglobin A1C): A blood test that measures the average level of blood sugar over 2-3 months

High-Intensity Interval Training (HIIT): A form of interval training, a cardio(vascular) exercise strategy alternating short periods of intense anaerobic exercise with less intense recovery period

Hormone Replacement Therapy (HRT): Medications given to replace hormones that decrease at the time of menopause

Human Papilloma Virus (HPV): A sexually transmitted virus that causes cervical cancer

Intrauterine Device (IUD): A birth control device placed in the uterus

Introital: Of or related to the opening of the vagina

In Vitro Fertilization (IVF): A fertility treatment that unites eggs and sperm outside of the human body and then places the fertilized egg in the uterine cavity

Kegels: Strengthening exercises performed on the Kegel, or pelvic, muscles

Mastopexy: A plastic surgery procedure to lift sagging breasts

Menarche: The age at which females start to menstruate

Menopause: The last menstrual period or end of reproductive life

Mirena: A progesterone containing IUD used for birth control or management of abnormal uterine bleeding

Molimina: Normal symptoms that occur between ovulation and menstruation that include breast tenderness, food cravings, fatigue, sleep problems, headaches and fluid retention

Myomectomy: A surgical procedure to remove fibroid tumors from the uterus

Nexplanon: A progesterone containing birth control device that is inserted in the arm

Nonsteroidal Anti-inflammatory Drugs (NSAIDs): A common pain reliever medication that is available by prescription and over-the-counter as aspirin (e.g., Bayer, St. Joseph), ibuprofen (e.g., Advil, Motrin) and Naproxen sodium (Aleve)

North American Menopause Society (NAMS): A society that promotes research and education on menopause

Oral Contraceptives (OCs) / Oral Contraceptive Pill (OCPs): Oral contraceptive pills, aka birth control pills

Osteoblasts: Cells that break down bone

Osteoclasts: Cells that build bone

Osteopenia: Thinning of the bones generally related to age but also due to various medications

Osteoporosis: Thinning of the bones that results in increased risk for fracture with minor trauma

Ovary: The female reproductive organ that produces eggs

ParaGard: A nonhormonal copper containing intrauterine device (IUD) used for birth control

Pelvic Inflammatory Disease (PID): An infection of the female reproductive organs, often including the uterus, ovaries and fallopian tubes

Perimenopausal: Also known as the climacteric, is literally the time "around menopause" or last menstrual period, which marks the end of the reproductive phase of life

Postmenopausal: When a woman has not had her period for an entire year and no longer produces estrogen in any meaningful amount

Premenstrual Dysphoric Disorder (PMDD): A severe form of PMS that causes life altering premenstrual and menstrual symptoms

Premenstrual Syndrome (PMS): Emotional and/or physical symptoms that occur prior to and during menstruation

Postpartum: After delivery

Pre-diabetes: A medical condition that is marked by elevated levels of glucose (blood sugar) that are not high enough to qualify as diabetes

Premarin: A type of hormone replacement therapy that is made from pregnant mares' urine

Premature Ovarian Insufficiency (POI): Early menopause

Premenopausal: Women in their later reproductive years, early to mid-40s, who are still having regular menstrual cycles

Progesterone: A female hormone

Prolia: A medication used to treat bone loss

Prometrium: A female hormone medication that is equivalent to progesterone

Pulmonary Embolism: Blood clot in the lung

Reclast: A medication used to treat bone loss

Selective Estrogen Receptor Modulators (SERMs): Medications that block the effects of estrogen in various body tissues

Soporific: Something that causes fatigue or sleepiness

Statins: A class of medications used to decrease blood cholesterol

Stress Urinary Incontinence: Involuntary loss of urine with abdominal straining

Thromboembolic Disease: Disorder that results in blood clots that break loose and travel to and block other blood vessels in the body

Testosterone: A male hormone

Uterine Artery Embolization (UAE): A radiologic procedure done to block blood vessels to uterine arteries to stop excessive bleeding and/or shrink fibroid tumors

Uterine or Endometrial polyp: A fleshy and usually benign growth in the uterine, or endometrial, cavity

Uterine Fibroids or Leiomyomas: Benign tumors made up of muscle cells and fibrous connective tissue

Vasomotor Symptoms: Hot flashes and night sweats

Vulvovaginal Atrophy: The medical term used to describe the thinning of vaginal and vulvar tissue prior to and after menopause

Women's Health Initiative (WHI): A study done in the 1990s to evaluate the effects of estrogen therapy on the prevention of heart disease

Works Cited

Admin. "Normal Ovarian Function." Rogel Cancer Center | University of Michigan, April 10, 2018. https://www.rogelcancercenter.org/fertility-preservation/for-female-patients/normal-ovarian-function.

The Editors of Encyclopaedia Britannica. "Hippocratic Oath," December 4, 2019. https://www.britannica.com/topic/Hippocratic-oath.

"Female Sexual Dysfunction." *Obstetrics & Gynecology* 134, no. 1 (2019). https://doi.org/10.1097/aog.0000000000003324.

Foley, Katherine Ellen. "Five Animals Experience Menopause. Four of Them Live Underwater." Quartz. Quartz, August 29, 2018. https://qz.com/1372767/twice-as-many-animals-go-through-menopause-as-scientists-previously-thought/.

Fraser, Ian S, Malcolm G Munro, and Hilary OD Critchley. "Abnormal Uterine Bleeding in Reproductive-Age Women: Terminology and PALM-COEIN Etiology Classification." UpToDate. Accessed May 9, 2020.https://www.uptodate.com/contents/abnormal-uterine-bleeding-in-reproductive-age-women-terminology-and-palm-coein-etiology-classification.

Hook, Ernest B., Philip K. Cross, and Dina M. Schreinemachers. "Chromosomal Abnormality Rates at Amniocentesis and in Live-Born Infants." *Jama* 249, no. 15 (1983): 2034. https://doi.org/10.1001/jama.1983.03330390038028.

"Life Expectancy." Wikipedia. Wikimedia Foundation, July 25, 2020. https://en.wikipedia.org/wiki/Life_expectancy.

National Osteoporosis Foundation. "A Guide to Calcium-Rich Foods" https://www.nof.org/patients/treatment/calciumvitamin-d/aguide-to-calcium-rich-foods/

"Practice Bulletin No. 141." *Obstetrics & Gynecology* 123, no. 1 (2014): 202–16. https://doi.org/10.1097/01.aog.0000441353.20693.78.

Watson, Stephanie. "Childbearing Age: What's Ideal and What Are the Risks?" Healthline. Healthline Media, June 6, 2018. https://www.healthline.com/health/womens-health/childbearing-age.

About the Author

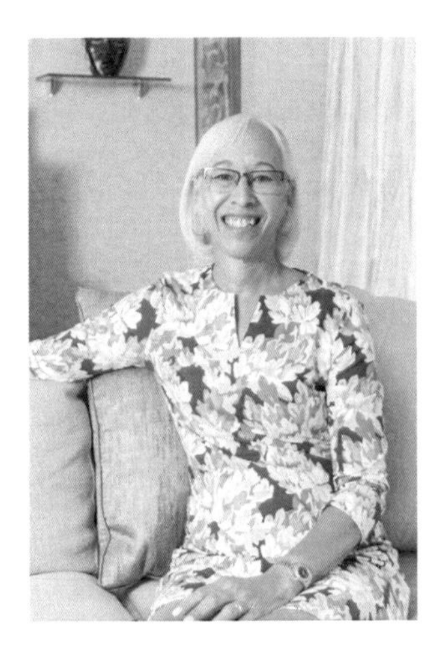

Dr. Heather Johnson is an actively practicing gynecologist and recently retired obstetrician after delivering babies for over 40 years. She is senior partner at Reiter, Hill & Johnson, an Advantia practice, with offices in Washington, DC, Chevy Chase, MD, and Falls Church, VA. She has been in private practice since 1987.

Dr. Johnson received her MD at Yale University School of Medicine and completed her residency training in obstetrics and gynecology at Walter Reed Army Medical Center, then located in Washington, DC. Dr. Johnson is board-certified in obstetrics and gynecology as well as a fellow of the American College of Obstetrics and Gynecology. She served in the US Army for eight years prior to going into private practice. She has two children and two grandchildren.

In her first book, *What They Don't Tell You About Having a Baby: An Obstetrician's Unofficial Guide to Preconception, Pregnancy, and Postpartum Life*, Dr. Johnson shares what she has learned throughout her career of over 40 years (delivering more than 3,500 babies) to assist parents and parents-to-be of all ages.

More information about Dr. Johnson and her books as well as her invaluable Dr. J's Pearls can be found on her website at https://askdrheatherjohnson.com/

She can be reached at writedrj@gmail.com and info@askdrheatherjohnson.com.